FRIENDS
IN HIGH PLACES

A Christian Guide To Fighting
And Overcoming Cancer

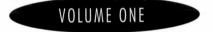
VOLUME ONE

Rev. Lillian Elizabeth Barnhardt-Israel

TATE PUBLISHING
AND ENTERPRISES, LLC

Published by Tate Publishing & Enterprises, LLC
127 E. Trade Center Terrace | Mustang, Oklahoma 73064 USA
1.888.361.9473 | www.tatepublishing.com

Tate Publishing is committed to excellence in the publishing industry. The company reflects the philosophy established by the founders, based on Psalm 68:11,
"The Lord gave the word and great was the company of those who published it."

Book design copyright © 2011 by Tate Publishing, LLC. All rights reserved.
Cover design by Sarah Kirchen
Interior design by Nathan Harmony

Published in the United States of America

ISBN: 978-1-61346-442-7
1. Health & Fitness / Healing
2. Health & Fitness / Diseases / Cancer
11.08.16

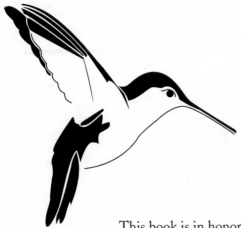

This book is in honor of my mother,
Ruth Magdaline Faith Thornton,
who was the first person to ever teach
me about the love of our
Lord and Savior, Jesus Christ. At eighty-
eight years old, she continues to teach me
His love daily and how to bring honor to His name!

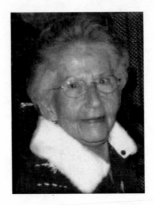

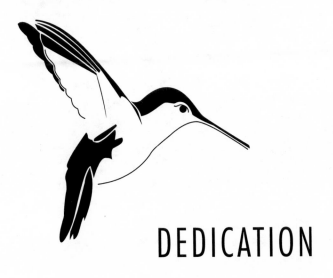

DEDICATION

There is a time for everything,
And a season for every activity under heaven:
A time to speak, and a time to build,
A time to love, and a time to heal...
Ecclesiastes 3:1 NIV

This F.R.I.E.N.D.S. Christian Cancer Care, Inc. guidebook is dedicated to you, the reader and participant, for your journey through cancer at this moment in your life.

The reason I chose the elegant beauty of the hummingbird for my front cover of this guidebook is because the hummingbird has many symbolisms attached to it, all of which are very positive. The ones that stood out to me as an author and cancer overcomer were the following:

A hummingbird symbolizes timeless joy and the Nectar of Life. It's a symbol for accomplishing that which seems impossible and will teach you how to find the miracle of joyful living from your own life circumstances. Did you know hummingbirds can't walk? But, they are the best flyers of all birds and fear no predators—they have even been seen driving off eagles! Hummingbirds are called new world birds because they are native to North America, Central and South America, and are considered to be symbols of peace, love and happiness. They are esteemed for their tireless energy and seemingly no anxiety. The colored ribbons the hummingbird is holding in her feet represent each type of cancer. She is flying as an overcomer to victory over all cancer!

Please know this is not an accident for you to be holding this F.R.I.E.N.D.S. guidebook at this time. It is God's plan and provision that you join us through the healing process for yourself and those who love you, as well as the medical professionals who will also accompany you on this journey. We, at F.R.I.E.N.D.S., believe God's word that states in Jeremiah 29:11:

> For I have a plan and purpose for your life that is good and filled with expectancy to bring you a future and hope. NIV

We also want to say how grateful we are for all those who had a part in shaping our lives and this F.R.I.E.N.D.S. Christian Cancer Care, Inc. guidebook through their tireless help and efforts to share these truths. We also want to thank God for the honor and privilege He has given us to share this with you!

—Rev. Lillian Elizabeth Barnhardt-Israel,
Cancer Overcomer
President/Secretary and Co-Founder of
F.R.I.E.N.D.S. Christian Cancer Care, Inc.

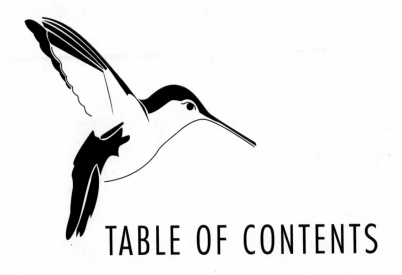

TABLE OF CONTENTS

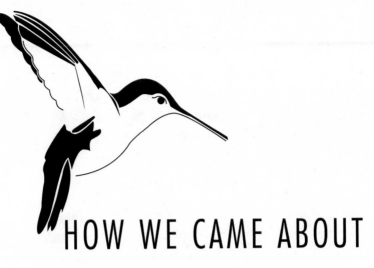

HOW WE CAME ABOUT

By Morris S. Dees, III, M.D.,
Oncologist, Vice President/Medical
Director and Co-Founder of
F.R.I.E.N.D.S. Christian
Cancer Care, Inc.

The summer before I went to medical school, I attended a lecture where I met a great Oncologist, George Selby, MD.

After the lecture, I spoke with Dr. Selby. He asked me if I wanted to attend his cancer clinics and help him take care of his cancer patients. It was then I knew exactly where I fit. It was like being at home.

I loved the intense relationships with these patients who were fighting for their lives. I also loved evaluating the rapid pace of new life-saving treatments I could help them with. However, I was puzzled why some patients with the same diagnosis did so much worse, while others were healed and had so much more peace in their cancer journey.

I prayed for the knowledge to help cancer patients in the way God wanted me to do. It is funny how some prayers are answered. I mistakenly walked into an office and met a radiation oncologist. She asked me to sit and talk. To my surprise, she said she was moving and asked if I would take over her cancer support group. Of course, the hair on the back of my neck stood up, and I said yes!

I had learned group therapy during graduate school for my master's degree in counseling psychology. During medical school, I went to the oncology floors in the hospital and asked patients to come to the support group.

It was there I found the answer to one of my prayers. A charming woman with leukemia would come to every group with her chemo pole in tow, which she called her "dancing partner." The effect she had on the group was profoundly uplifting.

Her peace was always evident, even though she was dealing with a deadly disease. I asked her how she had such serenity and she replied, "God is my physician and through Him I am healed."

Then and there, I knew that patients not only needed the very best medicine and medical care—they needed a spiritual focus as well! Again, I prayed to God to help me find a way to treat the whole person: the body, the mind, and the spirit. God listened and brought Rev. Lillian Elizabeth Barnhardt-Israel, a minister and breast cancer patient, to my office one day.

We prayed together for God to heal her and create something wonderful from her journey through cancer. I asked her to write a prayer for cancer patients. This led to F.R.I.E.N.D.S. Christian Cancer Care, Inc.

Our group is a special place where God's healing power touches us all. We feel His love as we laugh and cry together.

Now we want the world to know they have a place to come for God's comfort. We want everyone who is affected by cancer to know there is hope and peace through God's Holy Word. Come and help us as we help others.

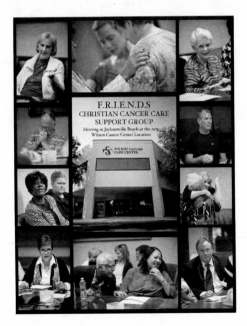

Rev. Lillian Elizabeth Barnhardt-Israel

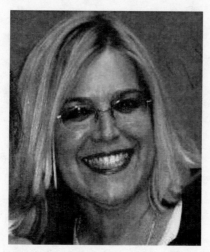

F.R.I.E.N.D.S. Volunteer Assistant

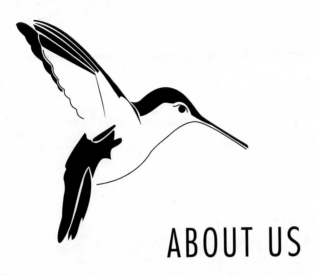

ABOUT US

By Rev. Lillian Elizabeth Barnhardt-Israel,
Cancer Overcomer,
President and Co-Founder of
F.R.I.E.N.D.S. Christian Cancer Care, Inc.

F.R.I.E.N.D.S. Christian Cancer Care, Inc. was born in my heart on April 4, 2006, when I was diagnosed with Stage 3C breast cancer. According to statistics, most cancer patients *do not live* five years with my diagnosis. After my surgeon discussed all my options and left the room, the surgical nurse assigned to my case continued to elaborate on my situation. She looked at my daughter and me with absolutely no expression in her face, and said, "You and your daughter need to be prepared that we are in the cutting out business-not the healing business-and your life will never be normal again!" All the air was sucked out of the room for Nicole and me. Needless to say, I knew my life was beginning to change forever.

The acronym F.R.I.E.N.D.S. stands for Friends Respond In Every Need Doing Something. My friends responding to my situation, in every need, with God's great compassion and love is exactly what took place during my battle with this terrifying and dreadful disease. In a very faithful and practical way, dear friends and family responded daily taking care of my challenging needs.

All of my family, including my only daughter, Nicole, lived out of town. From the very first moment of finding the cancerous lumps, my daughter and all of my friends sacrificed and prayed for me. It included many trips to the doctor's office with me to confirm the findings, biopsies, several surgeries, more doctor appointments, enduring radical chemo, radiation, and hospital stays in ICU. It also meant spending the night with me, grocery shopping for me, etc. You name it; God surrounded me with friends to help carry me through when I was too weak and sick to do it for myself alone.

My main hope and faith has always been in my Lord and Savior, Jesus Christ, to heal me and bring me through this season of nightmare. However, the love of God shown through my daughter, family members, pastor/employer, co-workers, plus the incredible care and excellence of the doctors and their staff gave me a confidence I was always among friends.

God gave me a peace from the very beginning of this journey with cancer that my course in this life was not finished. It was my only desire that I would bring honor to God during this time and take His hope everywhere this trial would take me. God assured me through my inner peace, and His Word, that He was going to take this hard and challenging time with cancer and make something beautiful out of it. He certainly did!

For me, after receiving the diagnosis, I was desperate to find a personal word from God that would sustain me and strengthen my heart. I went back to a scripture out of psalms my mother quoted over me all through my childhood.

> HE WHO dwells in the secret place of the Most High shall remain stable and fixed under the shadow of the Almighty [Whose power no foe can withstand]. I will say of the Lord, He is my Refuge and my Fortress, my God; on Him, I lean and rely, and in Him I [confidently] trust! For [then] He will deliver you from the snare of the fowler and from the deadly pestilence (malignant, deadly and devastating disease).
>
> Psalms 91:1–3 AMP

After reading this psalm that had been part of my life for years, the words *deadly pestilence* jumped out at me. As the Amplified version states, this phrase deadly pestilence means malignant, deadly and devastating disease. As a person who studies the Bible, it never occurred to me until that very moment in my life this spoke of cancer.

This understanding made me very aware that the answer for me to stay in peace and faith became very clear. If I was to be successful in fighting this horrific disease, I had to hide myself in the shadow of God's presence and declare daily God was my refuge and strength. I had to make a choice instead of letting the word cancer scream at me, that I had to lean on God and the faithfulness of His promise to me in His word that He would deliver me.

Every morning and at all times during the day and night, I prayed and quoted this psalm in the Holy Bible with my mom and daughter. God had brought me through so many trials of life, from losing my husband to every experience you can imagine, and He restored me fully. My hope was in God, but I soon found out the first week, I also needed my friends to help me, as I was too sick and weak to take care of myself alone.

On the very first visit to my oncologist, Morris S. Dees, III, MD, my daughter and I soon found out he was not your average doctor. Dr. Dees soon became not only my medical advisor but for Nicole and me, he became our close spiritual friend.

Dr. Dees had the exact same vision for healing through the power of Jesus Christ that Nicole and I knew to be true. Dr. Dees acknowledged that day, "I am just a vessel God uses and flows through, but God is the ultimate healer." We prayed together and discussed that the vital need for overcoming and managing cancer was spiritual well-being through a personal relationship with the Lord Jesus Christ. Dr. Dees asked me to write a prayer for cancer patients, which I did and it was copyrighted in 2006. It is called

The Prayer of a Doctor and a Patient. Thus, F.R.I.E.N.D.S. Christian Cancer Care, Inc. was officially born!

It was told to me by my Pastor and employer that my goal during this time should only be to get well. It was all my friends standing with me and helping me that allowed me to concentrate on the goal before me. It is now the most prominent desire of Dr. Dees and me to take this message to the medical community. We also desire to make this knowledge available nationally and internationally to all those affected by cancer, that our purpose statement which is, "Working together with the medical community for health and healing through faith and prayer" is not only possible but medically proven vital for overcoming and managing cancer. Our F.R.I.E.N.D.S. Christian Cancer Care, Inc. is making this possible! (For research reference please see www.friendsccg.com by Harold Koenig, M.D., of Duke University, Professor Psychiatry and Behaviorial Sciences.)

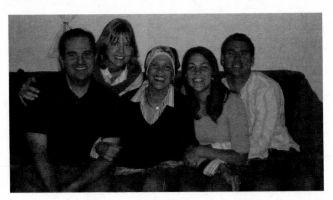

The Petrellos, Me, My daughter and Son-in-Law

THE PRAYER OF A DOCTOR AND A PATIENT

Together, as doctor and patient, Lord, we acknowledge You as Lord of our lives.

Together, we believe Lord; in You are absolute truth and all wisdom. We also acknowledge Your Word, in the Holy Bible, which declares there is no greater power than the prayer of unity.

Together, Lord, we therefore pray in unity and according to Your Word. We ask for Your wisdom, courage, and spiritual understanding. We also pray and ask for Your healing will in our bodies, hearts, and minds.

Together, Lord, we acknowledge that we will each do our part while trusting You to take care of all the rest.

We also acknowledge Your plan toward us, and our loved ones are good, and full of mercy, love, and kindness.

Together, Lord, we also acknowledge and trust You that You will never leave us nor forsake us, no never.

Together, Lord, during this journey, we pray believing that when we call upon You, we know You will hear and answer us; You will be with us in any kind of trouble, and that You will deliver us and honor our prayers.

Together, Lord, we declare there is no name higher than Your name, so in the precious name of the Lord Jesus Christ we pray. Amen.

—Rev. Lillian Elizabeth Barnhardt-Israel
Cancer Overcomer,
President and Co-Founder of
F.R.I.E.N.D.S. Christian Cancer Care, Inc.
Through the encouragement of
Morris S. Dees III, M.D., Oncologist,
Vice President/Medical Director and Co-Founder of
F.R.I.E.N.D.S. Christian Cancer Care, Inc.

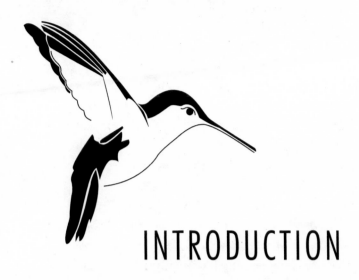

INTRODUCTION

By Rev. J. Stephen McCoy

Welcome to F.R.I.E.N.D.S. Christian Cancer Care, Inc.! You have begun a journey, either as a cancer patient, or as a friend or family member of a patient. Along with your expert medical care, we feel it is important for you to receive spiritual care too. This spiritual care will make the difference in your journey. Many of your fears and questions will find answers, and you will find peace and confidence.

All spiritual journeys have a beginning, and this one is no different. We must begin with a solid foundation. The Bible tells us there is only one way to align our hearts with God. This is through the sacrificial death and resurrection of His Son, Jesus Christ.

You may have been a Christian for many years, and you may have been in church all of your life. On the other hand, you may be someone who has had very little spiritual interest thus far in your life. Regardless, it is our desire for us all to begin this journey together, in one mind and one accord. We would like to ask you to pray the following prayer.

The Bible tells us that if you pray these words and believe the words you are speaking, that you will partake of God's fullest provision. You will receive help and grace now, and the promise of eternity for the future.

Join me now and let us begin our spiritual journey together by saying the following prayer:

> "Lord Jesus, we come to the throne of Your grace to receive grace to help in our time of need. We believe You are the Son of God and that Your Father sent You to earth. You came, You lived, You suffered, and You died for us. We believe You were raised from the dead and that You are alive for evermore. We ask You to forgive us for all of our sins and all of our trespasses. Please come into our hearts and be Lord of our lives. Thank You Lord Jesus. Help us to know You and to learn Your ways."

Let the journey begin. It is our prayer your passage will be with joy, great grace and comfort of the Holy Spirit. Let the following words of the Psalmist be yours as well.

The LORD is gracious, and full of compassion; slow to anger, and of great mercy. The LORD is

good to all: and his tender mercies are over all
his works.

Psalm 145:8–9 NIV

God's compassion for you is beyond question. Let Him
comfort you with His tender mercies today. May the Lord
richly bless you and keep you.

OUR MISSION AND
PURPOSE STATEMENT

F.R.I.E.N.D.S. gives comfort, spiritual support and benevolent assistance to those affected by cancer.

F.R.I.E.N.D.S. works in concert with the Medical Profession to promote good health and healing.

F.R.I.E.N.D.S. does this through the power of prayer, faith, and hope in monthly support group meetings, website interaction and personal ministry.

F.R.I.E.N.D.S. also provides benevolent and emergency assistance on a case by case basis.

Therefore, the purpose of F.R.I.E.N.D.S., in the following chapters, is to establish the need for spiritual help, prayer, and support. This allows the medical profession to work with the patient, family, and caregivers to handle the shock, dismay, and fear of the cancer diagnosis and the involved journey.

We ultimately look to God to take us through this trial. However, it is medically proven spiritual well-being is vital to overcoming and going through the process of cancer. (See Dr. Harold Koenig's, of Duke University, study on spiritual well-being on our website at www. friendsccg.com). F.R.I.E.N.D.S. is joining forces with the medical profession for health and healing through faith and prayer. Our focus is to bring hope during the trial of cancer and terminally related diseases.

—Board of Directors
Rev. Lillian Elizabeth Barnhardt-Israel,
Cancer Overcomer,
President/Secretary, and Co-Founder of
F.R.I.E.N.D.S. Christian Cancer Care, Inc.
Morris S. Dees, III, MD, Oncologist,
Vice President/Medical Director, and
Co-Founder of F.R.I.E.N.D.S.
Christian Cancer Care, Inc.
Archie O. Jenkins, III, Financial
Vice President, Treasurer of
F.R.I.E.N.D.S. Christian Cancer Care, Inc.
Haywood M. Ball, Esquire, Director of
F.R.I.E.N.D.S. Christian Cancer Care, Inc.
Rev. J. Stephen McCoy, Senior Pastor, Director of
F.R.I.E.N.D.S. Christian Cancer Care, Inc.

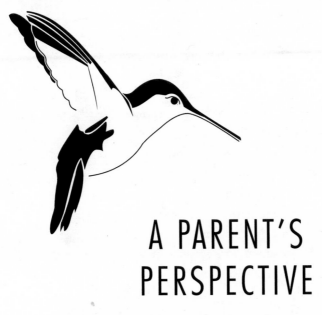

A PARENT'S PERSPECTIVE

Memorial to Haywood M. Ball, Jr.

Our son, Haywood M. Ball, Jr., was diagnosed with leukemia at age five. Our pediatrician sent us to the Jimmy Fund Clinic at Boston Children's Hospital for a confirming diagnosis. The doctor who advised us had a five-year-old child, and she gave us a plan in about twenty minutes, which we followed for the first year of Haywood's disease.

Since leukemia was such a frightening diagnosis and was considered terminal at the time, the doctor advised us to not call it by name but, she gave us another name in the anemia arena which I no longer recall. She said to explain that his disease was very serious and could be life threatening. This was to protect Haywood and enable him to have a normal life. I recall asking the doctor if she could prescribe something to help me sleep, and she refused saying I needed to face the situation.

Haywood was in remission for one year. From the outside everything appeared normal, but from the inside the silence was difficult because we could not talk to our family and close friends to explain what we were going through. Misleading people about Haywood's condition was not easy, but we matured as a couple having only each other for support and our wonderful doctors.

Unfortunately, a support group like F.R.I.E.N.D.S. Christian Cancer Care, Inc. was not available to us, and although our doctors were involved, they were not praying for us and Haywood.

When the cancer recurred, we were referred to Shand's Hospital in Gainesville, Florida, where the head of hematology had been trained at the Boston's Children Hospital. He explained that not all the doctors agreed with the advice given to us by our doctor in Boston. Therefore, this doctor encouraged us to tell our family and friends the truth. Our friends and family were supportive of our need to protect our son. However, it was a great relief to be able to share with them the situation and experience their love, support, comfort, and prayers for the next four difficult years prior to his death.

This experience is why I am so pleased to be a part of F.R.I.E.N.D.S. Christian Cancer Care, Inc. and the spiritual care and support they are able to provide patients and their families to manage and overcome cancer.

—Haywood M. Ball, Esquire
Director of
F.R.I.E.N.D.S. Christian Cancer Care, Inc.

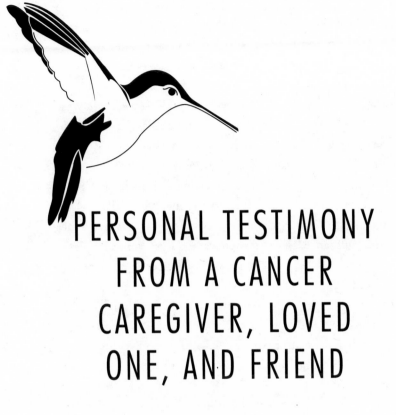

PERSONAL TESTIMONY FROM A CANCER CAREGIVER, LOVED ONE, AND FRIEND

It is an honor for me to be on the Board of Directors of F.R.I.E.N.D.S. Christian Cancer Care, Inc. because I have a personal vendetta with cancer, and how it has affected many of my family and friends through the years. It is very painful to see so many of my loved ones battling the many different types of cancers. Unfortunately, the list continues to grow.

One cancer battle I will never forget was of my Aunt Robin Jenkins. Aunt Robin lost her life way too young to cancer. If this particular type of cancer had been caught early, it could have been preventable. However, there was no support group other than her immediate family who also needed help to go through the challenges of this dreaded disease. Aunt Robin not only neglected her faith during this time, she remained isolated and withdrawn.

In my mind, the critical component F.R.I.E.N.D.S. Christian Cancer Care, Inc. creates is a *platform* that gives guidance, spiritual support, and direction. The platform of F.R.I.E.N.D.S. Christian Cancer Care Support Group also offers help and answers to the many questions that come with battling cancer. Most importantly, F.R.I.E.N.D.S. Christian Cancer Care, Inc. helps the patient fight cancer with their spiritual well-being combined with the physical well-being from the medical community.

This is a one-two punch affect that brings the healing power of God and the medical advances together for the very best combination. This insures the most successful and comforting journey possible through this trial. In my opinion, this is the best premise to cure cancer in a person's life.

I truly feel if Aunt Robin had gotten involved early in her cancer diagnosis with the Christian cancer care of F.R.I.E.N.D.S., Inc., she would be alive today. So my personal vendetta with cancer goes on, but in the future, I will make sure all my loved ones will be involved with F.R.I.E.N.D.S. Christian Cancer Care, Inc. Because

F.R.I.E.N.D.S. is a support team that brings hope and spiritual well-being, I am more optimistic than ever that we will know a time when all will be cancer overcomers!
—Archie O. Jenkins, III
Director of
F.R.I.E.N.D.S. Christian Cancer Care, Inc.

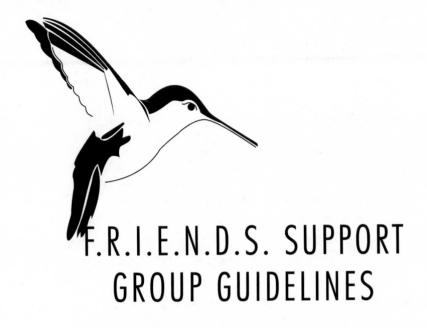

F.R.I.E.N.D.S. SUPPORT GROUP GUIDELINES

To keep our F.R.I.E.N.D.S. Christian Cancer Care, Inc. small group a safe place for everyone to share, we adhere to the following guidelines:

- We at F.R.I.E.N.D.S. believe in miracles, when things are impossible with man, all things are possible with God.

Jesus looked at them and said, "With man this is impossible but with God all things are possible."
Matthew 19:26 NIV

We are here to support one another, not "fix" each other. Please, there is *no* cross talk or trying to fix someone else with your personal suggestions. Cross talk is impolite and interrupts the individual processing their feelings and trying to communicate openly. Each person needs to be free to express his or her feelings without interruption.

Any personal, financial, housekeeping, or event needs are to be addressed outside of group time.

Support group time is a time for sharing our faith, hope, and support. This is not a time to seek personal medical advice or counsel from the medical professionals present at the meeting.

Go around and have each person share their first name.

The following is an explanation of the phases of the cancer diagnosis:

1. After receiving the diagnosis, "It is cancer," there are typically six phases: shock, denial, anger, bargaining, depression, and acceptance.

2. However, it does a great disservice to label one another at any given time so we can pigeon-hole where we all are in this process.

3. It is also a great disservice that we demand we all fit into neat little boxes and move through these phases sequentially. The phases are, in fact, seldom seen in a regular sequential order.

4. We may feel angry one day, depressed the next, and denying the next. And, the time frame may be a matter of hours and minutes.

5. It is better, therefore, to consider these phases tasks to be performed in no particular form or pattern, with no moral judgment determining which phases are "good" and which are "bad."

6. We will be discussing all the phases during our time together. We will apply the Word of God to each: alarm/shock; searching questions; despair/anger; ending in our identity/recovery and acceptance stages.

CHAPTER 1
Fear Versus Faith

Lesson Objective:

Overcoming Fear

Scripture Focus:

Romans 8:15–16   Fear is bondage. NIV
1 John 4:18   Knowing God's love for us
                         eliminates fears. NIV

Topic Discussion Question:

What has dealing with fear been like for you?

Suggested Prayer:

Father, I thank you that you did not give us a spirit of fear but you gave us by the Holy Spirit power, love, and a sound mind. Thank you, Lord, for faith arising in each of our hearts by the Holy Spirit of God to overcome and drive fear out during this challenging time of cancer. Amen.

Teaching:

How does fear versus faith relate to our diagnosis of cancer? We hear the word *cancer*, and immediately most of us experience fear in so many areas. We fear what will happen physically, mentally and financially. Our faith usually wavers weakly with the *"what if's."* What if I can't work, take care of myself or my family? What if I do not respond well to the treatment? What if I am alone or in pain? And the list goes on. If it is a family member who is diagnosed, there is a whole other set of questions and the *"what if's"* we deal with in our minds.

God wants to deal with all the core fears in each of us that are heightened by realizing we, or someone we love, has cancer.

The Lord wants to assure us that we do not have to be afraid of evil tidings that come with the knowledge of cancer. I found this to be personally true as I kept my heart fixed on God, as in the following psalm, instead of my situation.

> He shall not be afraid of evil tidings; his heart is firmly fixed, trusting (leaning on and being con-

fident) in the Lord. His heart is established and
steady, he will not be afraid while he waits to see
his desire established upon his adversaries

Psalm 112:7–8 AMP

No matter what our circumstances are surrounding deadly
diseases, God wants us to draw our strength from Him
and not be in fear. Why?

God wants to deal with our fears because fear and faith
cannot co-exist in the same heart. Fear is in direct opposi-
tion to faith. Fear capitalizes on the unknown in our lives.
Fear brings torment, especially when we are faced with
the critical news of a life-threatening illness.

When diagnosed with cancer, I was shocked, in dismay, and full of fears. For example, because I am a mid-
dle-aged widow, I heard lies screaming at my mind, such
as, *You will lose your hair and your looks,* and *nobody will
want you ever again. You will be disfigured–who will want
you then? You will be fired at work and end up in financial
ruin, all alone and in pain.* Lastly, no *one understands you
and they will all think you are too much trouble.*

All these fears were based upon a lie from the enemy,
the devil. He mixed it with a little truth to be convincing,
but it was still a lie. For me personally, I had to hold up the
truth of God's Word daily against these tormenting voices.

For example, the Word of God promises I will not be
ashamed that God will never leave me nor forsake me.
God also promises that He will take me through every
tribulation in this world because Jesus has already overcome the world's challenges. As I stayed in God's Word,

my mind stayed at peace and concentrated on getting well, not the *what if's*.

Every bit of faith is based on the truth of what God says in His Word such as the following scripture taking place in the Garden of Eden.

> Now the serpent, the devil, was craftier than any of the wild animals the LORD God had made. He said to the woman, to trick her, "Did God really say?"
>
> Genesis 3:1 NIV

The devil was craftier than any of the others. The devil has been speaking fear and using doubt by asking, "Has God said…?" since the beginning of time. Our part is to hold up the light of God's word to the devil's lie as shown in the following truth from the Book of James.

> Submit yourselves, then, to God. Resist the devil, and he will flee from you. Come near to God and he will come near to you.
>
> James 4:7–8 NIV

It became a stark reality that the more I knew of the Word of God, the more equipped I was to resist the attack of the devil and put down fear with the promises of God. The truth is, yes, I did lose my hair, but the lie was instead of people not wanting me, I had more people show God's love to me than ever before.

It has been my experience that we deal with the devil and all the fears he brings by taking the devil out of his element. The devil deals in darkness and lies. God deals in light and truth.

For example, if a shark is in the water, we get out of the water for fear of being attacked by the shark and getting hurt. But, if the same shark is in the parking lot, we are not afraid of him. Why? Because the shark is out of his element, which is the water. We are not afraid of him because he is on land where he cannot hurt us.

Holding the Word of God up to every fear the devil tries to frighten me with, I have learned it is absolutely necessary for me to expose that same fear to the light of God and His truth. This exposes the devil, who is now out of his element, which is darkness and lies. For me, speaking the following scripture out loud during these times of fear helped me find peace.

> Surely you desire truth in the inner parts; you teach me wisdom in the inmost place.
>
> Psalm 51:6 NIV

Fears are not a small issue, because many fears probably began earlier than we can remember in our childhood. Many of us, starting with infancy, lay up a storehouse of fears in our inward most parts. This takes place in our emotions and our imaginations. God has to deliver us from these fears.

The lie I believed was that I had to look perfect and be perfect for anyone to love me. In my going through Stage 3C breast cancer, having a double mastectomy, losing my hair and strength, God revealed to me the lie I was believing.

God took my fear of having to be perfect, and through my weakness, showed me that His love and strength was made perfect. This strengthened my trust in God.

Every fear that is exposed in our lives opens the door for the operation of faith in that place. Once we confront the fear, face it, and walk through it, we see we were not destroyed. We cannot change what we do not confront. Our faith in God to keep us continues to grow.

Knowing every fear is based upon a lie, we deal with the lie we believe and allow God through His Word to deal with the fear.

For example, "I fear man." I had to find a promise in God's Word that shed light and truth on this fear. Every time man has let us down, that experience will scream at us in a voice of fear not to ever again trust anyone. But, the truth is not every person alive is untrustworthy! As we walk with God, we learn we can trust people according to how much of the character of God is working in their lives. We become comfortable that our Lord will lead us in this area of trust.

> Fear of man will prove to be a snare, but whoever trusts in the LORD is kept safe.
>
> Proverbs 29:25 NIV

According to *Webster's II New College Dictionary*, the word *snare* means a trapping device, usually a noose, to entangle the unwary and cause them to stumble; to capture. As this relates to dealing with cancer, understanding that fear is a snare is most important because it will rob us of trusting God and others. As I found out, during this very personal and intimate time, I needed to be able to reach out and trust God and others greater than ever before in my life.

Personally, God had healed me, rescued me, and brought me through many physical challenges miraculously. I wanted God to do it the same way again: miraculously, with no surgery, or treatment. As I waited for the results of all the necessary medical tests, each time the results were confirmed, I was instructed that time was of the essence, and I needed to make decisions concerning my medical treatment. This was because I was already in Stage 3C of breast cancer.

Fear of man's capabilities had entrapped me, and I struggled in making treatment decisions in the beginning of my cancer journey. I was a widow and totally alone. The question I kept asking the Lord was, "Why not heal me again miraculously? Why do I have to suffer this invasive treatment with all these horrible side affects? How can I trust the capabilities of these men I do not even know?"

It was in a very personal moment with God on my front porch that the Lord spoke to my spirit: "Liz, you trusted me to save you and you submitted to the truth of my Word. You trusted your husband Bud when he was alive, and submitted to his authority. You have trusted and submitted to your pastor, as well as the men I have put in your life to give you advice and help you through Bud's death. Now Liz, I want you to submit your trust to the medical professionals I have surrounded you with, and believe that I will keep you through this process. Most of all Liz, remember I will never leave you nor forsake you. Most importantly, no matter what happens, do not forget I love you."

That afternoon, I was able to release my faith in God to keep me through the roller coaster ride of handling a terminal disease. I was able to submit and release my faith to trust the doctors God had brought into my life. Plus, they all turned out to be extremely well-qualified doctors, and more importantly, Christians!

Developing faith and releasing our fears to God, I have found is not a one-time event. Just as going through cancer is a process, so is seeking God and His truth over believing the devil and his lies. One of the scriptures I rely on to remind me that I have a responsibility to do my part in getting rid of fears is David's Psalm 34.

> I sought the LORD, and he answered me; God delivered me from all my fears.
>
> Psalms 34:4 NIV

This word *sought* means to seek, inquire of, search, study, investigate, and beat a path to daily.

In the Hebrew, "God delivering me from all my fears" means being delivered from a storehouse or a holding place. We do not even know what we are afraid of many times, or what we need but God always knows. For me to stay in faith while battling this deadly disease, I had to beat a path to God daily through His Word. Sometimes all I could manage to get out was, "Help Jesus, I am afraid. Jesus, I believe—help my unbelief!"

The Word of God became my closest friend as it brought clarity and power to separate what was confusing. I relied on the following verse from Hebrews much of the time.

> For whatever God says to us is full of living power: it is sharper than the sharpest dagger, cutting swift and deep into our innermost thoughts and desires with all their parts, exposing us for what we really are.
>
> Hebrews 4:12 TLB

Reading God's Word was vital for me. We all can be in denial about having fears and especially while in the presence of others. As believers, we think sometimes that even if we express our fear to God, we must be weak in our personal faith towards God. This is a lie the devil uses against us to keep us from coming boldly into God's presence in time of our trouble. We naturally want to withdraw when we are in fear. Fear can also open the door to self-pity, anger and rejection when we are sick or overwhelmed.

God is going to deliver us from all of our stored up fears as we seek Him and learn His Word. Only God knows what we fear, but God also promises that if we seek Him, He will deliver us as is stated in Hebrews 4:13.

> God knows about everyone, everywhere. Everything about us is bare and wide open to the all-seeing eyes of our living God; nothing can be hidden from him...
>
> Hebrews 4:13 TLB

As I sought God and gave myself to His Word, God emptied me of all of my fears. God filled those places I surrendered to Him with more of Himself; His glory, His presence, and His character in my life. Cancer may have taken a lot of things from me, but this is the one thing it could never take, and that is the security, love and peace I know in God.

> But Jesus the Son of God is our great High Priest who has gone to heaven itself to help us; therefore let us never stop trusting him. This High Priest of ours understands our weaknesses and fears.
>
> Hebrews 4:14–15 TLB

For me, knowing that Jesus understood my weaknesses and fears gave me hope. As I read the scriptures daily, faith overrode all my fears involving this disease. We all have a storehouse of fears that we store up over a lifetime, and they can become strongholds of fear in our lives. The word *stronghold* means an area occupied or dominated by the devil.

What is the answer for breaking free of these strongholds? We need to give ourselves to the Word of God every day and apply the truth of what God says every time fear wants to come against our hearts. God encouraged me through my battle with fear that I could come every day to His throne for His grace in time of my need as the following scripture describes.

> So let us come boldly to the very throne of God and stay there to receive His mercy and to find grace to help us in our times of need.
>
> Hebrews 4:16 TLB

Our prayer needs to be daily, "God, keep me from evil and in my heart show me where the pitfalls of the devil are when he tries to bring fear against me." For cancer patients, most of the time, the two greatest fears for us are: the fear of pain and the fear of being alone. God addresses these fears in His Word. Knowing these truths and reminding myself there was an answer in His Word for all the following fears kept me in faith, hope and peace.

The Bible speaks about the greatest areas of fear, in addition to the fear of man, as listed in the following:

1. Fear of Evil (or pain) and being alone:

> Even though I walk through the valley of the shadow of death, I will fear no evil, for you are with me; your rod and your staff, they comfort me.
>
> Psalms 23:4 NIV

> The LORD himself goes before you and will be with you; he will never leave you nor forsake you. Do not be afraid; do not be discouraged.
>
> Deuteronomy 31:8 NIV

As I hid Psalm 23 and Deuteronomy 31 in my heart, God revealed to me I had to choose daily between staying under the shadow of His presence or the shadow of death. When the shadow of death tried to hover over me like dark clouds of fear and confusion, I chose to speak out loud, "I know the cure for the fear of evil (or pain) and being alone is to know God will never leave me nor forsake me. God is with me no matter what my circumstances are in the midst of dealing with cancer and the possibility of death. I release myself from fear right now in Jesus' Name and choose to believe you, Lord, to take care of me."

2. Fear of Death:

> And deliver them who through fear of death were
> all their lifetime subject to bondage.
>
> Hebrews 2:15 KJV

Dealing with the fear of death, as believers in the Lord Jesus Christ, we know death is just a transition from this temporary world to an eternal life with Jesus Christ, Our Lord. We know death is just a step, a promotion to seeing Jesus face to face.

There is no fear or sting in death when we can know and believe this truth in God's Word. This is another truth I would speak out loud, pray, and give to God. Such peace would always settle over my heart as I quit living from test to test and surgery to surgery. Instead I would declare, "Lord, take this situation and turn it into something beautiful for your glory. As long as I am on this earth, I ask God that my days would count for you whether you heal me on this side of Glory or the Glory-side of Heaven!"

Also, in the midst of all my treatments, fear tried to grip my heart as I experienced all the physical changes, such as loosing my hair and watching it fall out right before me. It was terrifying at first, then depression wanted to overwhelm me. Fear during the trial of cancer robs us of a sound mind and clear thinking. The following scripture in Timothy became one I held close to my heart.

> For God hath not given us the spirit of fear; but of power, and of love, and of a sound mind.
>
> 2 Timothy 1:7 KJV

There will always be circumstances or someone that will scream, "This is a hopeless situation and you should just give up." But God wants to be the hope and strength of our hearts. God wants us to walk in the power and love of His Word with a mind at peace no matter what the circumstances are before you.

Fear has torment, but understanding the perfect love of God for us will set us free and keep us in peace. This has become part of life's journey for me. I found special comfort in the declaration from the Book 1 John.

> We need have no fear of someone who loves us perfectly; his perfect love for us eliminates all dread of what he might do to us. If we are afraid, it is for fear of what God might do to us and shows that we are not fully convinced that he really loves us. So you see our love for him comes as a result of his loving us first.
>
> 1 John 4:18–19 TLB

God promises to work all things for our good even the trial of cancer. Because of this challenge with cancer, F.R.I.E.N.D.S. Christian Cancer Care, Inc. was born. God truly took something horrible and turned it into something good that would bless and bring hope to the multitudes. It has become one of the most important things I can do, when a difficult situation arises, and that is to allow the scripture below to guide me and my thoughts.

> And we know that all things work together for good to them that love God, to them who are the called according to his purpose.
>
> Romans 8:28 KJV

In the course of our lives, we all have to decide, "Are we going to tremble in fear or choose to believe God and rise to faith?" With cancer, it is an ongoing process of choosing faith for today. The author of Hebrews describes what faith is in a very practical way.

> What is faith? It is the confident assurance that something we want is going to happen. It is the certainty that what we hope for is waiting for us, even though we cannot see it up ahead. Men of God in days of old were famous for their faith.
>
> Hebrews 11:1–2 TLB

It is my personal desire that we may all be known as men and women of faith today. In the days to come as together we walk through the challenge of cancer, it is also my desire, that we may be found trusting the Lord to keep us as described in the Book of Isaiah.

> When you pass through the waters, I will be with you; and when you pass through the rivers, they

will not sweep over you. When you walk through
the fire, you will not be burned; the flames will not
set you ablaze. For I am the LORD, your God, the
Holy One of Israel, your Savior.

Isaiah 43:2–3 NIV

Chapter 1—Summary of Fear Vs. Faith

Lesson Discussion: Overcoming Fear During the Battle
of Terminal Illness

Scripture Focus:

Romans 8:15–16	Fear is bondage NIV
1 John 4:18	Fear has torment NIV
Psalm 34:4	I sought the Lord and He delivered me from all my fears. NIV

Doctor's Comments:

When patients hear they have cancer, their whole world
changes. The word *cancer* is a shock and paralyzes their
minds. Time stands still and they cannot process any
further information. They ask, "Why me?" and "Has
God forsaken me?" God's Word has comfort for us and
removes our fears of annihilation. Seeking God's Word
daily throughout the journey of cancer will release you
from fear. God will also use this cancer diagnosis to get
closer to you. God wants you to know His love for you
and that you are healed in His love.

Topic Discussion:

How does the three basic fears: fear of evil (being alone, being in pain), fear of death, and fear of man affect your life?

Suggested Closing Prayer:

Father, I thank you that you did not give us a spirit of fear but you gave us by the Holy Spirit, a spirit of power and love and a peaceful mind. Thank you, Lord, for faith arising in each of our hearts through trusting the promises of Your word. Thank You, Lord, by Your great grace we can overcome and drive fear from our lives during this challenging time of dealing with cancer. In Jesus' mighty name. Amen.

Additional Follow-Up Scriptures:

✓ 2 Timothy 1:7	Fear robs us of a sound mind. NIV
Romans 8:28	God will work it for good. NIV
Revelation 12:11	They overcame by the blood of the Lamb. NIV
John 8:32	The truth will set you free. NIV
Psalms 56:3	When I am afraid, I will trust in you. NIV

Notes:

_____

_____

_____

_____

_____

_____

_____

_____

_____

_____

_____

_____

_____

_____

Rev. Lillian Elizabeth Barnhardt-Israel

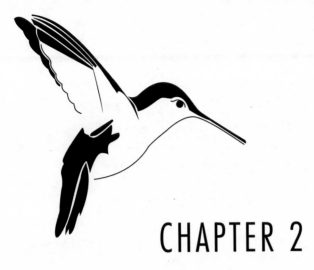

CHAPTER 2

Why Me—Does God Really Love Me?

Lesson Objective:

Is God punishing me with sickness, and how does it relate to the diagnosis of cancer?

Scripture Focus:

Isaiah 53:7 NIV God paid the ultimate penalty

Topic Discussion Question:

Why me—does God really love me?

Suggested Prayer:

Lord, we thank you for your everlasting love toward us. God, thank you that you loved us so much you gave your only son, Jesus, that we would be free from sin, sickness and death; to know your love and spend all eternity with you. Lord, we ask for a greater revelation of just how much you love us—change our hearts to receive all that you have for us today and every day. In Jesus' Name. Amen.

Teaching:

Man is three parts: spirit, soul, and body.

When we are born again, our spirit is justified and made perfect. We are at peace with God. Our soul is our intellect, feelings, emotions, and heart. Our soul is being renewed in a knowledge of God daily. Our body is the last to be redeemed in the process of salvation and ultimately resurrection. Therefore, from the day we are born, our bodies are in a process of deterioration. Living beyond three score and ten years (or seventy) is grace.

In the resurrection, our bodies are made perfect and we receive eternal bodies. In our glorified bodies, we will not be affected with sickness, disease, aches, pains, or cancer. This in no way negates God's ability to heal but the ultimate healing is in eternity with Him.

These are very important truths we need to be well founded in, know and remind ourselves often of especially when sickness strikes our lives. King Solomon talks about the importance of acknowledging God in all our ways even in illness. This allowed me to accept and trust that

God was going to make my path straight even though at times I felt the road was a very rocky and winding place.

> Trust in the LORD with all thine heart; and lean not unto thine own understanding. In all thy ways acknowledge him and he shall direct thy paths.
> Proverbs 3:5–6 KJV

When we are confronted with the finality and mystery of death, we are prompted to ask many questions that only Scripture can answer. To answer the statement, "I am terminal, and I am going to die," can be answered, "We are all terminal."

> And as it is appointed unto men once to die, but after this the judgment.
> Hebrews 9:27 KJV

Death is not an end: death is a beginning. Our eternal life with God begins when we are born again and continues through death and through eternity. What does it mean to spiritualize events in our lives such as physical illness?

It means every circumstance, event, cause of nature, or human behavior is attributed to a spiritual sense or meaning. For example, if I pull out in front of moving traffic, I will be hit by another car. It was my choice, and a bad choice. To spiritualize the car accident would be to say God or the devil made me pull out.

To jump off a building onto concrete three stories below will definitely hurt you. It is the law of nature. If I make a choice to jump off this building, I will fall below onto concrete. Even if I say, "I will jump off because God spoke to me," I am not going upward, I will fall downward. I can spiritualize it and attribute my broken body to God, but it was because I made a choice against the law of gravity and suffered the consequences.

Therefore, we cannot spiritualize or attribute cancer to God or judge someone who is sick that they deserved to get sick. Physical bodies are designed to wear out after a certain amount of years.

The Scriptures declares, "It is appointed once for every man to die."

> Just as man is destined to die once, and after that
> to face judgment.
>
> Hebrews 9:27 NIV

To spiritualize sickness and how we die is to take every human being's destiny and demand God give us answers. When we don't get those answers, there is only one result: we get angry with God. Rather than spiritualizing, we need to acknowledge God in all our ways.

We must make a choice to believe and receive God's promise that He loves us. It is a natural reaction when diagnosed with cancer to confront a variety of confusing thoughts, reactions, and conclusions. We think, *Is God mad at me? What did I do to bring this on myself?* Or we point fingers and judge others who are sick. This is spiritualizing the diagnosis of cancer. This is wrong.

How many times, when your children were really bad, did you ever wish cancer on them? Never!

When we spiritualize and ask, "Why me and why did God allow this? Doesn't God love me?" This is wrong because our temporary earthly bodies were not meant to live forever. Our body from the moment we are born is in a state of decay. Sometimes our bodies break down early and unexpectedly. It is our human nature to grieve at the loss of our loved ones, especially when it seems they go before their time.

> The righteous perisheth, and no man layeth it to heart: and merciful men are taken away, none considering that the righteous is taken away from the evil to come.
>
> Isaiah 57:1 KJV

These bodies just wear out. We don't reach eighty years old without some things just breaking down in our physical bodies. It is not practical or realistic for us to think we would last forever. Our bodies will just give out for many natural reasons in this life.

With the diagnosis of cancer, in the midst of this confusion, we usually ask ourselves, "Do I deserve this?" or "Is the purpose of my life over and has God forsaken me?"

In my first week alone after surgery and in the beginning of my treatments, I lost my hair and strength right away. Friends had to move my bed downstairs so I could reach the kitchen and bathroom.

There were so many experiences where fear wanted to totally grip my heart and paralyze me. However, the vastness of being totally alone and helpless became a reality I had never experienced. I was blessed with a strong physical body and strong optimistic belief that things would always work out. This particular night around 3:00 am, my body failed me and I couldn't move my legs. I was gripped with fear. My body was also crashing into the side affect of neutropenia where my temperature would spike with fever and then hit a low with shaking chills.

The only strength I had was to roll out of bed onto the floor. I was on my face before God and I cried out to Him with what little voice I had left. "God, if I have to go through this, somehow turn it for good and use it for your glory." It was a time of being terrified and weak. The Lord spoke to my heart and said, "I have plans for you and your course is not finished." Peace came over me and I was able to pull myself up to the bed and I slept for a couple of hours. When I awoke, God gave me the "The Prayer of a Doctor and a Patient" plus the entire plan for F.R.I.E.N.D.S. Christian Cancer Care, Inc. Throughout the last five years, I have clung to the Word of God and remembered God still had a plan for my life.

> "For I know the plans I have for you," declares the LORD, "plans to prosper you and not to harm you, plans to give you hope and a future. Then you will call upon me and come and pray to me, and I will listen to you. You will seek me and find me when you seek me with all your heart. I will be found by you," declares the LORD, "and will bring you back from captivity."
>
> Jeremiah 29:11–14 NIV

God delivered me from the captivity of fear and wondering if I had done something to deserve this disease moment by moment, day by day, week by week. It has now been five years after that night where I felt my life was over. God has shown me that where there is no vision the people perish. We can still each have purpose and passion through His Word even lying in our beds sick and weak. God wants us to be convinced of His love towards us and His plan for our lives.

For me, cancer truly was a situation to open new doors of divine relationships and divine plans for my life. God did not give me cancer anymore than I would have caused my child to have cancer, but He used this frightening challenge and turned it into something wonderful.

Our behavior and thinking is influenced by our understanding of God's love for us. We ask, "Is God punishing me with this sickness?" Nothing could be further from the nature of God. He loves us and wants us delivered from the lie, and the fear, that He does not love us.

> "As the Father has loved me, so have I loved you. Now remain in my love."
>
> John 15:9 NIV

For me, realizing the truth of God's love kept me from feeling like I had done something wrong to deserve this horrible disease. This continually sets me free from any condemning voices the devil would try to scream at me. In my personal relationship with God and struggling with the trauma of cancer, it was vital I knew the difference between what it meant to have this disease because of many reasons - or to spiritualize the situation and blame myself or God. When we try and spiritualize our circumstances with cancer, we attribute things to God in which He has had no part.

There are a variety of reasons why we can have cancer: There is our ever-changing environment, our genetic makeup, and our hereditary traits. They all figure into our physical makeup, both good and bad. God does not afflict His children with sickness to teach them lessons or punish them. Jesus came that that we would have and enjoy this life to the fullest!

> The thief comes only to steal and kill and destroy;
> I have come that they may have life, and have it
> to the full.
>
> John 10:10 NIV

Further, when we spiritualize and blame God for our condition with cancer, we fall into a trap, which will keep us from partaking of God's best for our lives.

During this time of trouble and pain, one of the scriptures that meant so much to me was the promise of Jesus that whatever I face, He has already made a provision for me to overcome that trouble. My responsibility was only to believe, and that would keep me in perfect peace.

> "I have told you these things, so that in me you
> may have peace. In this world you will have trouble. But take heart! I have overcome the world."
>
> John 16:33 NIV

Chapter 2—Summary of Why Me— Does God Really Love Me?

Lesson Discussion:

Is God punishing me with sickness?

Scripture Focus:

Isaiah 53:7 NIV God Paid the Ultimate Penalty

Doctor's Comments:

Many patients say, "But I didn't smoke or do anything in excess. I exercised and did everything right." As an oncologist, I hear that all the time. One patient, a young woman with Hodgkin's disease, felt God was punishing her for her lack of faith and mistakes she had made. She felt she had not been a good mother as her children were leading unsuccessful lives. She was so distraught with guilt; she initially chose to have no treatment for a highly curable cancer. She even stated, "I would rather die." This patient was angry, arguing with our staff and nurses to the point that she was nearly fired from our practice. In fact, she was depressed. With counseling, I suggested she was to focus on God's enduring love for her. She finally accepted her treatment and is cancer free now for five years.

Topic Discussion Question:

How has learning that God loves you and is totally for you, and your healing, changed your perspective of the cancer diagnosis? What is your biggest challenge in believing God loves you?

Suggested Closing Prayer:

Lord, we thank you for your everlasting love toward us. God, thank you that you loved us so much you gave your only son, Jesus, that we would be free from sin, sickness and death; to know your love and spend all eternity with you. Lord, we ask for a greater revelation of your love. In Jesus' Name. Amen.

Additional Follow-Up Scriptures:

Isaiah 53:7	God paid the ultimate price NIV
John 8:32	The truth will set you free NIV
Jeremiah 31:33	God's everlasting covenant NIV
Ephesians 3:14–20	God wants us to experience His love NIV
Psalm 100:3	God's love endures forever NIV

Notes:

_____

_____

_____

_____

_____

_____

_____

_____

_____

_____

_____

_____

_____

_____

Rev. Lillian Elizabeth Barnhardt-Israel

CHAPTER 3

How Do I Handle the Anger?

Lesson Objective:

Anger steals our strength and joy. The Word of God is the Lord's remedy for handling anger and returning our joy.

Scripture Focus:

Proverbs 12:25	An anxious heart weighs a man down NIV
Nehemiah 8:10	Great mirth because they understood the words NIV

Topic Discussion Question:

What makes you angry and causes you to lose your joy? Why do you think it is important to keep your joy?

Suggested Prayer:

God, the fruit of righteousness is peace and joy, without being anxious or angry no matter what the circumstances. Help us, Lord, through your great grace to give you every care, concern, anxiousness and all anger so that we might stay in joy and peace each day. In Jesus' name, Amen.

Teaching:

Being angry opens the door of our hearts for the devil to have his way in our lives.

> If you are angry, don't sin by nursing your grudge. Don't let the sun go down with you still angry-get over it quickly; for when you are angry, you give a mighty foothold to the devil.
>
> Ephesians 4:26–27 TLB

While I had to handle the practical every day demands of life while I was so sick, I always asked the question to myself, "In the light of eternity, is this particular situation worth getting all upset over, or is it better for me to make the choice to just let it go and give it to God."

God wants us in peace. Being angry over our circumstances keeps us upset. The devil's goal is to steal our joy so we will lose even more strength when we are sick. Our goal, or the goal of a caretaker, is to use our strength to manage the challenges of every day with balance and peace. For me, I had to learn I can only do this by remembering the promise of God through His covenant with me.

> Therefore tell him I am making my covenant of peace with him. He and his descendants.
>
> Numbers 25:12–13 NIV

Are you angry? It is normal to be frustrated and upset, but God does not want us stuck in this painful place. Anger can actually bring us more physical discomfort through stress in our bodies.

Anger is one of the most common emotions when diagnosed with cancer. Once our fears wane slightly, it is natural to become angry with God and with others because we have been, or someone we love has been diagnosed with this devastating disease.

Common questions of exasperation are: What about my plans? What about my physical looks and relationships? What about my loved ones? Unfortunately, these are difficult questions to answer, so the tendency is to become frustrated, and then angry.

How do we overcome this anger?

Each day I found my questions were answered as I walked with God through the days of my diagnosis, surgeries, treatment, and care. It was my experience of having a solid foundation of God's promises to me in His Word that I was able to be an overcomer during this battle with cancer. This foundation was absolutely vital to my spiritual well-being.

What do I do when my mind is whirling with angry and fearful thoughts?

> The weapons we fight with are not the weapons of the world. On the contrary, they have divine power to demolish strongholds. We demolish arguments and every pretension that sets itself up against the knowledge of God, and we take captive every thought to make it obedient to Christ.
>
> 2 Corinthians 10:4–5 NIV

To overcome trouble and anger, we must daily seek and read the Word of God.

> You will keep in perfect peace him whose mind is steadfast, because he trusts in you. Trust in the LORD forever, for the LORD, the LORD, is the Rock eternal.
>
> Isaiah 26:3–4 NIV

It was also very important for me to surround myself with people of like faith who could encourage me in the Lord daily, especially when I was feeling overwhelmed.

> Whatever is true, whatever is honest, whatever is just, whatever is pure, whatever is lovely, whatever is kind, if there is any virtue, if there is anything worthy of praise, think on these things.
>
> Philippians 4:8 NIV

We know that anger is one of the most common emotions known to mankind. Without anger, there would be no passion. In fact, hardly anything of any value would ever get done without the passion against injustice.

One of the benefits of being trained in God's word is that we are aware that redirected anger is what can drive us as individuals to do great things in God. It becomes righteous indignation against injustice, evil, and the devastating works of the devil. This happened to me personally walking through this affliction and suffering with cancer.

> Be self-controlled and alert. Your enemy the devil prowls around like a roaring lion looking for someone to devour. Resist him, standing firm in the faith, because you know that your brothers throughout the world are undergoing the same kind of sufferings. And the God of all grace, who called you to his eternal glory in Christ, after you have suffered a little while, will himself restore you and make you strong, firm and steadfast.
>
> 1 Peter 5:8–10 NIV

Important Note: When we talk about controlling our anger, we speak of anger management and not anger elimination.

We all experience anger, but managing our anger is crucial during the time when we are under pressure and especially when we are overwhelmed or sick.

God wants us to manage our anger in a way that is productive and not destructive. You might be saying to yourself, "I cannot seem to control my anger." As believers in Christ, we can—starting right now!

We have all had the experience of being in the midst of an argument when our phone rings. We go from raising our voices to being calm and saying hello. This is anger management. It is a choice we make daily, and at times moment by moment.

Knowing what the scriptures have to say about anger will help us to be better managers of our anger.

> Those who control their anger have great understanding; those with a hasty temper will make mistakes.
>
> Proverbs 14:29 NLT

Anger is a God-given emotion, and sometimes anger is the most appropriate emotion, especially when we see people hurt, taken advantage of, being cheated, or abused. Anger is also a normal emotion when we have been given a shocking diagnosis that will change our lives forever, and the lives of the ones we love.

In fact, if we never get angry, it could be an implication that we have never loved strongly or we are in denial of our feelings. Being honest before God daily and communicating our feelings is the safest way to recognize and deal with our frustrations.

We must learn to control our anger, to use it wisely, and to manage it. When we get angry, we tend to clam up or blow up, but neither is managing our anger in a way that is useful. When we are faced with circumstances that are completely out of our control, I found the more I could keep my mind on the promises of God and not keep repeating my frustrations over and over, I was able to manage my emotions.

> A [self-confident] fool utters all his anger, but a wise man holds it back and stills it.
>
> Proverbs 29:11 AMP

Staying angry or holding back is a choice. Because I can always choose to get angry or not, therefore, I can always choose to control my anger. The Bible says there is a cost for all uncontrolled anger.

It has been my experience that I am less likely to get angry if I can remind myself that there is a cost for my anger. Notably, it is always a price tag I am not able to afford. We need to reflect before we get angry because anger is almost always an impulsive reaction. I have found if I can control my tongue, I can begin to control my anger. Anger management is very practical: it is largely mouth management and what we allow to come out of our mouths.

Suggested Tools for holding back our anger are:

- Think before we speak. Delay is a great remedy to anger. We need time to cool down.

We should not delay expressing what made us want to act in anger, because our communication needs to be clear. The Bible says, "Do not go to bed angry." Carrying anger over to the next day without open communication often causes deeper resentment. I personally have found this true; have you?

What are some positive steps we can take once we start becoming angry?

- I can step back and ask myself truthful questions such as: Why am I angry? Why am I getting so upset? Why am I feeling this way? What is my goal and objective, and when compared to all of eternity, does this really matter?

- I can examine my heart and see if I have gotten my feelings hurt. Most of the time we get angry when we are hurt, devalued, or rejected. If I recognize I am hurt, I can be open and honest to communicate this hurt to the person who hurt me rather than getting angry myself. This is my responsibility. Their responsibility is to respond appropriately without anger as well.

Especially when dealing with illness, anger can also be caused by frustration because we are trying to control the uncontrollable either in people or our circumstances. The only thing we have control over is our own response and behavior.

Jesus told us the following in Isaiah 26:3:

Thou wilt keep him in perfect peace, whose mind is stayed on thee: because he trusteth in thee.

Isaiah 26:3 KJV

If I can take a moment and consider this scripture I will realize if my mind is not at peace, then it is a good indication my actions are not being led by Jesus.

It has been noted that high control people are also high anger people. It is a good question to ask ourselves when we feel frustrated: What am I trying to control that is out of my control?

It is a wonderful realization once we acknowledge most things are out of our control in this journey called life. Then we can accept what we cannot change, and pray for the courage to change what we are able to change. Acceptance that Jesus is in control brings great peace as we give our frustration to Him.

We can also note that when we get angry, many times the anger is rooted in fear. Jesus was also very clear about the spirit of fear.

> For God hath not given us the spirit of fear; but of power, and of love, and of a sound mind.
>
> 2 Timothy 1:7 KJV

So many times during the process I had to go through, I would get frustrated because I felt I was held hostage or cornered by tests, medicine and the daily regimen. We all know that when you corner a wild animal, most often they will come out fighting and roaring. It is much the same with human beings. When we feel cornered, we want to come out fighting. Fear causes us to lose control of our emotions, and we start to get anxious, insecure, and threatened, and eventually this can result in anger, if we do not deal with the fear and the cause of our fear.

What is the appropriate way to handle our anger? The following are a few things I have learned:

- Only God can handle vengeance—we must hand our anger over to God. The Webster's II New College Dictionary defines *vengeance* as the act of punishing another in payment for wrong doing or injury.

- Don't give voice to the anger, because the more we say things and discuss it, the angrier we become.

- Step back and pray. Try to consider and decide if this is something so important that I should be angry about? Then make a conscious decision to give it to the Lord and release control of the situation. Make a choice and resolve within yourself to do good whenever possible. For our own peace, do it even if it is to someone who has done evil to you.

- Lastly and above all, depend on God totally to diffuse you through prayer, communicating with God before railing on a person and read God's Word until you are at peace.

Beloved, never avenge yourselves, but leave the way open for [God's] wrath; for it is written, Vengeance is Mine, I will repay (requite), says the Lord.

Romans 12:19 AMP

As human beings, we cannot handle vengeance. God knew this and reminded us over and over how important it is for us to stay clear and in peace. The more we stir up anger, the angrier and more stressed out we stay. This is harmful to us in every way—body, mind, and spirit.

> And let the peace (soul harmony which comes) from Christ rule (act as umpire continually) in your hearts [deciding and settling with finality all questions that arise in your minds.]
>
> Colossians 3:15 AMP

What does this mean if I lose my peace, and when I am provoked to anger? It means the situation that was on the outside of me, to cause me anger, is now raging on the inside of me. We need to keep the storm out of our lives by keeping the storm in its proper place and perspective.

I can remain at peace when I refuse to believe that my life is under the control of anyone other than God. For example, Paul was a prisoner, but he acknowledged only God could have allowed the situation for a reason. Therefore, Paul was not a prisoner of Rome but only a prisoner to the will of God, and that kept him in perfect peace no matter what situation Paul found himself in.

This is why I can remain at peace even through the battle with cancer. Because no matter what my circumstances in are, God promises to take every situation and work it for my good if I will acknowledge Him.

> And we know that all things work together for
> good to them that love God, to them who are the
> called according to his purpose.
>
> Romans 8:28 KJV

In the above verse, God is talking about you and me as believers in Christ. Whatever the state of our affairs, if we can acknowledge God in all our ways, God will work it to our good. We may not see it now, but as we go through and look back over other trials we came through, we can see how God took ashes and made something beautiful in our lives.

Chapter 3—Summary Of How Do I Handle The Anger

Lesson Discussion:

"How do I handle the anger of what cancer is doing and has done to me, emotionally and physically?"

Scripture Focus:

> Thou wilt keep him in perfect peace, whose mind
> is stayed on thee: because he trusteth in thee.
>
> Isaiah 26:3 KJV

Doctor's Comments:

A woman I saw a year and a half ago had a recurrence of breast cancer. Her lungs filled with fluid, and she had tumors. After getting to know her, I could see her anger toward her daughter was going to be a major obstacle in her treatment and recovery as well as with her relationship with God. During our initial interview, she told me about her ungrateful, embarrassing daughter's behavior.

I was unable to complete my medical evaluation. Her bitterness was palpable. It was easy to see it had come between her and her husband. Certainly the stress of her relationships weakened her immune system response and hindered her recovery response with cancer.

We spent many hours talking about forgiveness. We prayed together to begin the process to forgive her daughter. There was a lightness to her heart, and it was evident she had a happiness. She also had a positive response to treatment and was cancer free after her first cycle of treatment. Unfortunately, forgiveness is something we have to ask God's help to accomplish and maintain individually. Then I noticed she began talking and denigrating her daughter again, and her scans indicated a return of cancer. It became more difficult for her to get well because she was so bitter.

Topic Discussion Question:

Anger is one of the most common emotions known to mankind. Without anger, there would be no passion. In fact, very little, of any value, would ever get done against injustice with the passion of anger. Do you agree with this?

It has been noted, losing our health is the same process as when we lose someone we love. It is the same grieving process. Anger at what is happening in our lives can sometimes surprise us. We find we are in an emotional roller coaster. Have you found this to be true?

Suggested Closing Prayer:

Heavenly Father, we thank you for your peace during these very anxious and stressful times. You told us there would be tribulation in the world but not to worry because you have overcome all that is in the world that can hurt us and rob us of peace. Come and be our comfort and our peace in Jesus' name. Amen.

Additional Follow-Up Scriptures:

Proverbs 14:29	Those who control their anger have understanding NIV
Proverbs 29:11	A [self-confident] fool utters all his anger NIV
Proverbs 29:22	An angry man stirs up dissension NIV
Romans 12:19	Beloved, never avenge yourselves NIV
Colossians 3:15	And let the peace from Christ rule in your hearts NIV
Isaiah 26:3	Thou wilt keep him in perfect peace, whose mind is stayed on thee NIV

Notes:

_____

_____

_____

_____

_____

_____

_____

_____

_____

_____

_____

_____

_____

_____

Rev. Lillian Elizabeth Barnhardt-Israel

CHAPTER 4

Eternal Reward

Lesson Objective:

Why even go through all of this? Why not give up?

Scripture Focus:

| Matthew 14:28 | Peter said, "If it be Thou you Jesus, bid me to come." NIV |
| Matthew 11:28–30 | Learn of me … and you shall find rest. NIV |

Topic Discussion Question:

As believers in Christ, we are building eternal reward through every challenge of life. Even though we know this, aren't we all a little like the Bible character Peter experiencing roller coaster emotions?

Suggested Prayer:

Lord, you say learn of Me and we shall find rest. We ask for greater faith and the rest that can only come from leaning on You. In Jesus' name. Amen.

Teaching:

No matter what we say or do, Jesus loves us and is the anchor of our soul. Many times I forgot this and thought I did not measure up, but Peter's example always reminds me it is God's faithfulness to bring me through, not my faithfulness.

A good picture of our roller coaster faith is out of The Book of Matthew. This is when Peter who was compulsively brave ended up sinking with fear.

> "Lord, if it's you," Peter replied, "tell me to come to you on the water." "Come," he said. Then Peter got down out of the boat, walked on the water and came toward Jesus. But when he saw the wind, he was afraid and, beginning to sink, cried out, "Lord, save me!"
>
> Matthew 14:28–30 NIV

Isn't that just like us? Jesus speaks to us, and we say, "Yes, Lord." Then we are aware of all that is going to be involved, and we sink with all the circumstances surrounding us. Especially when we are trying to look really strong for our family members or loved ones while going through surgeries and treatments, but inside we are full of doubt, dread and fear!

> Immediately Jesus reached out his hand and caught him. "You of little faith," he said, "why did you doubt?"
>
> Matthew 14:31 NIV

Jesus had to remind Peter, just like He has to remind us, "Fear not. Do not worry, I am the Lord of all, even over nature and all practical issues of your life and I am with you. I will never leave you nor forsake you!"

It has been my experience when everything is going well and that means there is enough money in the bank, I am not feeling sick and plus all my relationships are in peace, then I am a lot braver. When I am sick or dealing with financial stress plus people problems and money being tight, I am certainly less brave. How about you? So our question should be, "Who and what are we really putting our faith in?"

Dealing with the heart wrenching decisions daily that came from all the changes in my life from being pronounced with Stage 3C cancer, there were times when I was so close to the Lord. His presence overshadowed me instead of the *shadow of death*. God revealed His love, protection and comfort greater than ever before. This I believe is what Peter experienced in his personal conversation with our Lord Jesus.

> Simon Peter answered, "You are the Christ, the Son of the living God." Jesus replied, "Blessed are you, Simon son of Jonah, for this was not revealed to you by man, but by my Father in heaven."
>
> Matthew 16:16–17 NIV

With all the ups and downs during this season in my life, it always encouraged me to consider Peter and his up and down faith. God loved Peter and called him "friend." With all of Peter's impulsive behavior, God saw through all of that to Peter's heart. This helped me fight the voices of condemnation when I could not be of practical value to anyone else, and my heart was breaking from the loneliness and isolation of the disease. God just loved me, whether I was able to give or perform for Him or not.

What a comforting promise. Because Jesus knew Peter's true heart as expressed in Matthew 5:37, Jesus chose to only let Peter follow him when he needed to pray for a healing miracle.

> He did not let anyone follow him except Peter...
>
> Mark 5:37 NIV

We are guilty of being like Peter when the difficulties and devastation of cancer hit us. We too, want to ask, "What then Lord, when I served you so faithfully?

> Peter answered him, "We have left everything to follow you! What then will there be for us?" Jesus said to them, "I tell you the truth, at the renewal of all things, when the Son of Man sits on his glorious

> throne, you who have followed me will also sit on
> twelve thrones, judging the twelve tribes of Israel."
>
> Matthew 19:27–28 NIV

We all believe we love the Lord with our whole hearts until we are faced with pain and suffering. It is in this moment of intense suffering, we each find out who we really are inside. God never reveals this to condemn us but bring us to a place of humility and trust where we say, "God you are right, and I am wrong. Please have mercy on me and overshadow me with your grace to go through this battle."

> Peter replied, "Even if all fall away on account of you,
> I never will." "I tell you the truth," Jesus answered,
> "This very night, before the rooster crows, you will
> disown me three times." But Peter declared, "Even if
> I have to die with you, I will never disown you."
>
> Matthew 26:33–35 NIV

However, when the chips are down, many times we are shocked at our thoughts and behavior of fear. Many times we are lost in the midst of the trial with cancer, and it breaks our heart, but Jesus understands us.

> For we do not have a high priest who is unable to
> sympathize with our weaknesses, but we have one
> who has been tempted in every way, just as we are—
> yet was without sin. Let us then approach the throne
> of grace with confidence, so that we may receive
> mercy and find grace to help us in our time of need.
>
> Hebrews 4:15–16 NIV

In the end, Peter was found faithful and obedient. After Jesus arose from the dead, all Peter could remember is how he failed Jesus. However, one of the first things Jesus told Mary after His resurrection was, "Go get Peter!" Sometimes when we are hurt or afraid, we wimp out and lose our faith in the face of adversity. But, Jesus knows our suffering and He looks on our hearts. By the Holy Spirit of God, He comforts us and draws us back to Him.

> Then Simon Peter, who was behind him, arrived and went into the tomb. He saw the strips of linen lying there, as well as the burial cloth that had been around Jesus' head.
>
> John 20:6–7 NIV

> And he saith unto them, Be not affrighted: Ye seek Jesus of Nazareth, which was crucified: he is risen; he is not here…
>
> Mark 16:6 KJV

We need to be settled and sure in our eternal reward with Jesus. This is a vital truth to understand. It does not matter what we have done, what situation Jesus had to bring us out of, or how many times we lost faith, God loves us.

> May they be brought to complete unity to let the world know that you sent me and have loved them even as you have loved me.
>
> John 17:23 NIV

God's whole plan is to save us body, soul, and spirit and for us to end up with the greatest reward possible for the life we have lived. Even during our challenges with this devastating disease, we are building reward in God.

Sometimes our reward is something we cannot measure in monetary value, like relationships, character, peace, a fresh sense of purpose, favor with others, clearer understanding and more compassion and intimacy with Jesus.

> To him who is able to keep you from falling and to present you before his glorious presence without fault and with great joy—to the only God our Savior be glory, majesty, power and authority, through Jesus Christ our Lord, before all ages, now and forevermore! Amen.
>
> Jude 24–25 NIV

Chapter 4—Summary Of Eternal Reward

Lesson Discussion:

Why even go through all of this? Why not give up?

Scripture Focus:

Hebrews 4:15   For we do not have a high priest who is unable to sympathize with our sickness and infirmities. NIV

Doctor's Comments:

Giving up is not just an issue for cancer patients but also for oncologists. I learned a valuable lesson from a patient who has become my teacher. This patient had ovarian cancer and had at least seven prior chemo regimens for her incurable disease over several years. Her previous Gynecologic Oncologist told her there was nothing more he could do for her when she was hospitalized for a pulmonary embolism and recommended hospice. When I saw this woman of great faith and her three young grandchildren she was raising alone, I too wondered what I really could offer. She exhorted, "Do not give up on me Doctor. I am all my babies have. Only God knows how long I have. In my heart I feel I am not finished." We began treatment and she immediately responded. Her CA-125 dropped, her tumors shrank, and thus she was able to care for her children. I pray to never forget her and her faith that God's will for her was all that she needed.

Topic Discussion Question:

When is it the most difficult, for you, to really care that we are building reward in God?

Suggested Closing Prayer:

Lord, in the midst of our pain and suffering, it is hard for us to remember that you understand and are with us every moment. Your Word declares you sympathize with us and pour out your grace and mercy in time of need. Thank you that You are changing us from strength to strength and glory to glory. In Jesus' Name. Amen."

Additional Follow-up Scriptures:

Matthew 16:16	You are the Christ, the Son of the living God NIV
Mark 8:29	Then "Who do you say I am?" NIV
Matthew 17:1	Jesus as friend and confidant NIV
Matthew 26:33	When we are faced with pain and suffering NIV
Matthew 11:28–30	Learn of me…and you shall find rest NIV

Notes:

_____

_____

_____

_____

_____

_____

_____

_____

Rev. Lillian Elizabeth Barnhardt-Israel

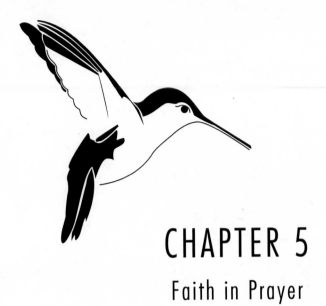

CHAPTER 5

Faith in Prayer

Lesson Objective:

Faith in Prayer

Scripture Focus:

James 1:6–8	A double minded man is unstable in all his ways. NIV
Hebrews 11:6	God rewards those who diligently seek him. NIV

Topic Discussion Question:

Is cancer my new identity? Or does God really want to reward me by giving me purpose and passion during this time? Why or why not?

Suggested Prayer:

Lord, thank you that every time we come to you in faith, you will carry us over, our faith pleases you; that your name is Faithful and True, and we can trust You. We love you, Lord, and release our faith to pray according to your word and your will. In Jesus' name. Amen."

Teaching:

Faith is the essential element in our prayer life. Without faith and confidence toward God in our prayers, we are actually begging God, and we have all been in that place. For many of us, it was all we knew to do.

Sometimes that is where our faith level is, but that is not the standard God has for us. God is not impressed with the eloquence of our words. God hears our prayers, because we have humbled our hearts before Him and drawn close to Him in the midst of our trouble and pain of cancer.

God looks at our hearts. God is after our whole heart to trust Him and His promises in His Word, the Holy Bible. We pray and communicate with God, because He is our source. God wants to shine His light and hope in every situation, even in the dark places of terminal illness.

The devil always wants us to doubt that God hears us and cares about us. Even though God is our source and we know it, we are still challenged to believe and are surprised when He answers our prayers.

For me, reminding myself of the story of Peter in prison, and how the saints of God were able to pray for him and he was delivered out of that place is amazing. However, even though they prayed, they really did not believe God heard and would act on those prayers.

> So Peter was kept in prison, but the church was earnestly praying to God for him.
>
> Suddenly an angel of the Lord appeared and a light shone in the cell. He struck Peter on the side and woke him up. "Quick, get up!" he said, and the chains fell off of Peter's wrists. Then the angel said to him, "Put on your clothes and sandals." And Peter did so. "Wrap your cloak around you and follow me," the angel told him. Peter followed him out of the prison, but he had no idea that what the angel was doing was really happening; he thought he was seeing a vision.
>
> Acts 12:5–10 NIV

There were sixty-four soldiers watching Peter who was bound with two chains. Herod intended to bring Peter out for public trial after the Passover. Just think of this fact again, four squads of guards were watching Peter, and he was bound by two chains. What a tremendous miracle for Peter to be able to walk out of this prison through prayers of the saints!

> They passed the first and second guards and came
> to the iron gate leading to the city. It opened for
> them by itself, and they went through it. When
> they had walked the length of one street, suddenly
> the angel left him.
>
> Acts 12: 10 NIV

We do not know if Peter was translated or made invisible, but his escape was supernatural! This is totally amazing, and that is how God wants us to look to Him when we are walking though the tough trial of sickness. God wants us expectant instead of always being so shocked when He does hear our prayers and answers them.

> Then Peter came to himself and said, "Now I know
> without a doubt that the Lord sent his angel and
> rescued me from Herod's clutches and from every-
> thing the Jewish people were anticipating." When
> this had dawned on him, he went to the house of
> Mary, the mother of John, also called Mark, where
> many people had gathered and were praying. Peter
> knocked at the outer entrance, and a servant girl
> named Rhoda came to answer the door. When she
> recognized Peter's voice, she was so overjoyed she
> ran back without opening it and exclaimed, "Peter
> is at the door!"
>
> Acts 12:11–14 NIV

Peter was standing right before them, and they still could not believe God had answered their request. Isn't that just like our reaction as God walks us through this Valley of the Shadow of Death? God keeps us at peace, as we go from surgery to surgery and test to test, doctor appointments and all of it. God hears all our prayers and we are always amazed when they are answered.

> "You're out of your mind," they told her. When she kept insisting that it was so, they said, "It must be his angel." But Peter kept on knocking, and when they opened the door and saw him, they were astonished. Peter motioned with his hand for them to be quiet and described how the Lord had brought him out of prison. "Tell James and the brothers about this," he said, and then he left for another place.
>
> Acts 9:15–17 NIV

They faithfully prayed for Peter, but they still were astonished to see that God had actually delivered him. Sometimes, we feel we deserve to be sick, and it is hard for us to believe God hears our prayers and requests much less answer them!

> I wait for you, O LORD; you will answer, O Lord my God.
>
> Psalms 38:5 NIV

Seeing angels in biblical times, during the first century church, was obviously common place and occurred often. Angels come in response to our prayers, as in the example of Peter being freed from prison by angels.

> For it is written: "He will command his angels concerning you to guard you carefully; they will lift you up in their hands, so that you will not strike your foot against a stone."
>
> Luke 4:10–11 NIV

Angels are a reality and angels are very much a part of God's plan to bring us peace and help in time of need.

> The LORD has established his throne in heaven, and his kingdom rules over all. Praise the LORD, you his angels, you mighty ones who do his bidding, who obey his word.
>
> Psalms 103:19–20 NIV

Consider angels when you pray. Angels harken to the Word of God. The angelic forces gather strength when we pray God's Word. Think of the times you have escaped a terrifying situation and there was no way in the natural you could have survived. Many times, we all have escaped death, and angels have helped us without us even knowing they were present.

According to the Scriptures we are not to give up praying when we do not see the answer right away, because God is always working behind the scenes in our behalf.

> And he said unto me, O Daniel, a man greatly beloved, understand the words that I speak unto thee, and stand upright: for unto thee am I now sent. And when he had spoken this word unto me, I stood trembling. Then said he unto me, Fear not,

Daniel: for from the first day that thou didst set thine heart to understand, and to chasten thyself before thy God, thy words were heard, and I am come for thy words.

Daniel 10:11–12 NIV

When we are in the middle of the intense circumstances of illness, we think our prayers are not being heard, but God promises otherwise. The angel tells Daniel, "I left the minute you began to pray." However, it took the angel twenty-one days to get to Daniel, because of warfare in the heavenlies from the devil's demonic forces from Persia.

But the prince of the kingdom of Persia withstood me one and twenty days: but, lo, Michael, one of the chief princes, came to help me; and I remained there with the kings of Persia.

Daniel 10:13 KJV

The prayer of faith always changes things and brings peace, even in the worst of circumstances. God wants us to believe and trust Him at His Word. God wants us to press through praying in faith until we know we have felt and seen a breakthrough.

Many times we stop praying because we get in unbelief, especially when we are frail and weak in our bodies through cancer. God wants us to press through to the end because He promises that His Word goes forth and never returns without results, as experienced by Daniel.

> Then the one who seemed to be a man touched me again, and I felt my strength returning. "God loves you very much," he said; "don't be afraid! Calm yourself; be strong-yes, strong!" Suddenly, as he spoke these words, I felt stronger and said to him, "Now you can go ahead and speak, sir, for you have strengthened me."
>
> Daniel 10:18–20 TLB

We do not know exactly what goes on in spiritual battles; however, we are guaranteed we have spiritual weapons to which we can fight with for results as Paul explains to us in Corinthians.

> The weapons we fight with are not the weapons of the world. On the contrary, they have divine power to demolish strongholds.
>
> 2 Corinthians 10:4 NIV

We know the devil and his demons are the prince of the power of the air. As instructed by Paul, we are called to press through this demonic contention and fight with prayer with the spoken Word of God. The angelic forces gather strength through our prayers. Michael the archangel came as Daniel prayed. This is true for us today as the disciple John declares in the New Testament.

> This is the confidence we have in approaching God: that if we ask anything according to his will, he hears us. And if we know that he hears us—whatever we ask—we know that we have what we asked of him.
>
> 1 John 5:14–15 NIV

God wants us to pray in faith toward Him, even as we want our own children to ask us in faith and believe we are trustworthy to honor their requests.

Chapter 5—Summary Of Faith In Prayer

Lesson Discussion:

How does knowing that God hears and answers prayer, affect how we feel about our own self worth as everything changes around us through illness?

Scripture Focus:

Acts 12:1–16 God is our source for everything NIV

Doctor's Comments:

A highly educated female patient who was also a very gifted writer had a brain tumor. This woman was highly respected for her intellectual capacity. She found she was not the same person after surgery and radiation for her malignant brain tumor. She was in her fifties. Her memory was not as sharp. She was aware of her loss of what she most esteemed—her intellect.

She struggled to find other worth. My prayer was always for her to see herself as made in God's image. Her depression deepened and she isolated from her friends. It was a sad spiraling down to an annihilation of her family. Unhappily, she had not accomplished all she wanted to do, which is not unusual for women of that age.

Unfortunately, she never found a place of faith, peace, or acceptance.

It is vital for patients to continue their spiritual journey and their relationship with God. I hope this lesson, "We are made in God's image," will bring you peace and the healing God intends for you!

Topic Discussion Question:

Is cancer my new identity, or does God really want to reward me by giving me purpose and passion during this time?

Suggested Closing Prayer:

Lord, thank you that every time we come to you in prayer, You are faithful to hear and answer us. We ask for a greater gift of faith to know this is true. We trust You and acknowledge You in all our ways. In Jesus' name. Amen."

Additional Follow-Up Scriptures:

1 John 5:13–15   This is the confidence that God hears us and will answer us... NIV

Notes:

_____

_____

_____

_____

_____

_____

_____

_____

_____

_____

_____

_____

_____

_____

_____

_____

_____

Rev. Lillian Elizabeth Barnhardt-Israel

CHAPTER 6
Faith In Speech

Lesson Objective:

Faith in speech

Scripture Focus:

Proverbs 18:21

Death and life are in the power of the tongue. NIV

Hebrews 10:23

Hold fast the profession of our faith. NIV

Topic Discussion Question:

Does it matter what we say while we struggle with failing health? Think over your words in the last twenty-four hours. Are they words of life or death to you and your situation? What can you do differently?

Suggested Prayer:

"Father, give us your grace to guard our hearts and our speech during this time. We pray that we would only speak words of life to ourselves and to others about our situation; not denying the facts nor the pain but believing your word that You desire healing for all of us. In Jesus' name. Amen."

Teaching:

How many of you have a problem with what you are saying, especially in overwhelming and difficult times?

> My dear brothers, take note of this: Everyone should be quick to listen, slow to speak and slow to become angry.
>
> James 1:19 NIV

Maybe you have heard also, God gave us two ears and one mouth. Do you think He was trying to hint to us? I personally had to take this scripture to heart when hit with all the information about physical changes to my appearance after surgeries, treatment and side effects, as well as the long term process I was facing.

My natural response was to talk about all the things that were negative and getting ready to happen to me. I felt out of control totally and had to fight the need to just "tell it all" to those who would listen.

The following scriptures were ones I would read in the beginning daily when bombarded with too much information to even process. I found the more I talked about the details the more I wanted to cry and give up, so I had to possess my soul through the Word of God. The Bible declares even a fool is counted wise when he holds his peace and does not give an opinion on everything. The Bible also encourages us that God has a season and timing for all things.

> A time to tear and a time to mend, a time to be
> silent and a time to speak.
>
> Ecclesiastes 3:7

Timing in God is everything ... I have found. During severe testing especially, we all have an opinion on what should be done and how it should be done right now! Constantly, I was reminded of the scripture of how only God's plan for my life will stand sure-no matter what I was facing.

> There are many devices in a man's heart; neverthe-
> less the counsel of the LORD, that shall stand.
>
> Proverbs 19:21 KJV

The Bible is saying all our decisions should be filtered through the Word of God and by the Holy Spirit of God. God leads us by our peace.

> Grace and peace to you from God the Father and
> the Lord Jesus Christ.
>
> 2 Thesselonians 1:2 NIV

Especially during the shock and confusion as I navigated through cancer, I needed to remember God wants to give us a supernatural peace through Him, and His guidance.

> Peace I leave with you; my peace I give you. I do not give to you as the world gives. Do not let your hearts be troubled and do not be afraid.
>
> John 14:27 NIV

It was at times when I would be troubled or afraid, I had to keep reminding myself, "Liz, it is important what you are saying during this time to yourself and others." When we are trusting God and at peace, then out of our mouths will come words of healing and life, but when our hearts are full of bitterness, anger, or unforgiveness, the words out of our mouths are just the opposite of everything God stands for. James, the brother of Jesus, has some very strong words concerning our speech.

> If anyone can control his tongue, it proves that he has perfect control over himself in every other way. We can make a large horse turn around and go wherever we want by means of a small bit in his mouth. And a tiny rudder makes a huge ship turn wherever the pilot wants it to go, even though the winds are strong.
>
> James 3:2–4 NIV

James is saying our mouths control our overall direction in life. When we are hurting, we tend to be self-centered and expecting everyone to understand why we are caustic in speech. However, this is a time we need to even have greater watch over what we say. Self-pity is expressed through our speech, and is very subtle. It certainly tried to grab a hold of me at times. Self-pity will always raise its ugly head when others want to know how we are doing. I prayed to recognize self-pity, and stop it in its tracks before anything came out of my mouth that would hurt myself or others. I found the more I would allow self-pity to have entrance in my conversation, the worse I would feel instead of better.

> So also the tongue is a small thing, but what enormous damage it can do. A great forest can be set on fire by one tiny spark. And the tongue is a flame of fire. It is full of wickedness, and poisons every part of the body. And the tongue is set on fire by hell itself and can turn our whole lives into a blazing flame of destruction and disaster.
>
> James 3:5–6 TLB

James is telling us that we start things in motion we cannot stop once the words are out of our mouths. We need to be very careful that we put the right words into motion. I knew I needed to speak truth about my situation and what my needs were, but I also became very aware of how what I said concerning my disease could worry others. This was especially true of those who loved me most.

My description of what I was facing or had gone through could really hurt my precious family and friends.

> The tongue has the power of life and death, and those who love it will eat its fruit.
>
> Proverbs 18:21 NIV

A lot of times, we put words into motion out of fear, and Jesus told us not to fear; He gave us power over fear with love and a sound mind! When we are afraid, our minds go many places and our mouths follow. God wants us to acknowledge Him in all our ways. Trust Him and fear must leave, because now we are in faith. For me, learning to recognize fear helped me to lean on God's Word immediately by reciting out loud verses like the ones below.

> Trust in the LORD with all your heart and lean not on your own understanding; in all your ways acknowledge him, and he will make your paths straight.
>
> Proverbs 3:5–6 NIV

> When I am afraid, I will trust in you.
>
> Psalms 56:3 NIV

As we acknowledge God, even when things do not make sense, He will take ashes and make something beautiful, even suffering through cancer. I am a living testament of that promise!

> … to give unto them beauty for ashes, the oil of joy for mourning, the garment of praise for the

spirit of heaviness; that they might be called trees of righteousness, the planting of the LORD, that he might be glorified.

Isaiah 61:3 KJV

Personally, I have found that as my mind is centered in on Christ and His faithfulness to me, my mouth will line up with words of faith and truth.

It gave me great joy to have some brothers come and tell about your faithfulness to the truth and how you continue to walk in the truth. I have no greater joy than to hear that my children are walking in the truth.

3 John 3–4 NIV

Why do we need to guard our mouths and hearts especially during such a hard illness as cancer? This is because God wants our hearts clear and at peace. When we murmur and complain constantly, it goes into our spirits and makes us feel worse.

It is at those most difficult times of loneliness and dismay that I found I had to cry out to God as my source and comfort. The Psalms became a great source of strength for me through the years I struggled with cancer. I remembered God promised me the joy found in the living water of His Word and flowers for comfort as I stumbled through the wilderness of this unknown territory called Stage 3C Breast Cancer.

My flesh and my heart faileth: but God is the strength of my heart, and my portion for ever.

Psalms 73:26 KJV

For the LORD is good and his love endures forever;
his faithfulness continues through all generations.

Psalms 100:5 NIV

Chapter 6—Summary Of Faith In Speech

Lesson Discussion:

Why the Lord gave us two ears and one mouth.

Scripture Focus:

Proverbs 18:21   Death and life are in the power of the tongue. KJV

Doctor's Comments:

I am remembering a patient who had endometrial cancer. It was a rainy day with lightening and thunder. She was initially told that she would die and that treatment would be futile. This was told to her by her initial oncology physician that her case was futile and she would die despite any efforts. Her tone was negative and she was angry. She could not get that physician's words out of her mind.

Those words became her words. She had fitful sleep, dreams, and was clinically depressed, sedentary, and had neglected her physical appearance. My prescription for her was a scriptural exhortation of the following. These words came to me for her, "God's love, peace, joy, and power are in everything I do." I wrote it on a prescription for her.

In the days and weeks ahead, she struggled with this assignment and often forgot it, but through encouragement I could see a real change in her spirit. She had many years of quality of life responding to various therapies and made such progress in her spiritual journey that her final days were ones of great peace.

Topic Discussion Question:

Does it matter what I am saying during this time?

Suggested Closing Prayer:

Father, give us your grace to guard our hearts and our speech during this time that we would only speak words of life to ourselves and to others about our situation; not denying the facts nor the pain but believing your word that you healed them all! In Jesus' name. Amen.

Additional Follow-Up Scriptures:

Proverbs 19:21	There are many devices in a man's heart; nevertheless the counsel of the LORD, that shall stand. KJV
Proverbs18:21	Power and life is in the tongue. KJV
Proverbs 3:5	Trust in the Lord with your whole heart. KJV

Notes:

_____

_____

_____

_____

_____

_____

_____

_____

_____

_____

_____

_____

_____

CHAPTER 7

Transformed into God's Character

Lesson Objective:

Transformed to God's Character

Scripture Focus:

Psalm 63:1   Early will I seek Thee. NIV

Philippians 3:10   That I may know Him. NIV

Topic Discussion Question:

What keeps you from seeking the Lord regarding your cancer? When is your best time with God?

Suggested Prayer:

Lord, you say taste and see the Lord is good, and blessed is the man who finds refuge in Him. Lord, we seek you and you alone to make all the crooked places straight in our lives. We are trusting you and you alone. In Jesus' name. Amen.

Teaching:

David wrote Psalm 63:1, a Psalm of David, when he was in the Desert of Judah. The Bible says he was a man after God's heart, yet his heart knew great distress in this psalm as he was pursued by his enemies in a wilderness.

During the trial of cancer, the best and dearest of God's saints and servants can feel like their lot has been cast in a wilderness place. This wilderness speaks of being lonely and solitary: desolate and afflicted, wanting, wandering, and unsettled and in a place of loss not knowing what to do with themselves.

It is in the wilderness place that we go from leaning on our own strength and learning to lean on the true strength of Jesus. For many of us going through cancer, surgeries, and treatments, we find for the first time we are not able to do everything in our own strong will and strength. God wants to rescue us when we are in that place of total weakness and surrender. As David cried unto the Lord in Psalm 63, I found myself in this place many times declaring, "It is true Lord no matter what happens, your love is better than life."

> O God, you are my God, earnestly I seek you; my soul thirsts for you, my body longs for you, in a dry and weary land where there is no water. I have seen you in the sanctuary and beheld your power and your glory. Because your love is better than life, my lips will glorify you. I will praise you as long as I live, and in your name I will lift up my hands. My soul will be satisfied as with the richest of foods; with singing lips my mouth will praise you. On my bed I remember you.
>
> Psalms 63:1–6 NIV

You might be asking yourself, "Why do I need to study the Word of God while going through the cancer trial? Why is spiritual well-being so important?" The Book of Galatians answers that question.

> But when the Holy Spirit controls our lives he will produce this kind of fruit in us: love, joy, peace, patience, kindness, goodness, faithfulness, gentleness and self-control.
>
> Galatians 5:22–23 TLB

Dealing with our cancer makes us realize our vulnerability and how our lives are but a vapor, the Word of God declares. This became a very big reality for me.

> Why, you do not even know what will happen to-morrow. What is your life? You are a mist that appears for a little while and then vanishes. Instead, you ought to say, "If it is the Lord's will, we will live and do this or that."
>
> James 4:14–15 (NIV)

When we get discouraged, above all times, we need to press into the Word of God. It is usually then I want to just withdraw and isolate, especially when I didn't feel well. During illness and hardship is when God wants us to trust Him the most. We are either going forward in our faith toward God or we are drawing back. There is no coasting in God. It helped me to remember when I meditated in Hebrews just how important this is to God.

> Now the just shall live by faith: but if any man draw back, my soul shall have no pleasure in him.
>
> Hebrews 10:38 KJV

The Word of God comes to show us what is really in our hearts. It is not to show everyone else; it is to show us. Aren't you glad? We cannot change what we are not willing to confront. God already knows what is in our hearts. The Word of God reveals to each of us attitudes that can be hidden as shown again in Hebrews.

> For the word of God is living and active. Sharper than any double-edged sword, it penetrates even to dividing soul and spirit, joints and marrow; it judges the thoughts and attitudes of the heart.
>
> Hebrews 4:12 NIV

God wants our hearts lined up with His Word for our own protection and spiritual well-being. Many times at night, when I was weak and tired, I would lay my Bible on my chest opened to a favorite scripture to encourage me like the one out of Proverbs.

> My son, keep your father's commands and do not forsake your mother's teaching. Bind them upon your heart forever; fasten them around your neck.
>
> Proverbs 6:20–21 NIV

Our *neck* in Hebrew means our will. God is saying to bind the Word of God to your will and let the Word of God guide you, especially in times of great challenge and fear.

> When you walk, they will guide you; when you sleep, they will watch over you; when you awake, they will speak to you.
>
> Proverbs 6:22 NIV

This became so important for me to do daily. I had to speak out loud that the plans of God would stand firm forever, as David declared in the Psalms. As the days became weeks and then years, I became more convinced the Word of God will always give us a plan through the darkest hours and circumstances in our lives.

> But the plans of the LORD stand firm forever, the purposes of his heart through all generations.
>
> Psalm 33:11 NIV

Knowing the Word of God is the only way to keep our hearts at peace and to do God's will. Through experience, I learned I cannot do what I do not know.

> ...guide me in your truth and teach me, for you are God my Savior, and my hope is in you all day long.
>
> Psalms 25:5 NIV

God gave us the written Word of God printed on a page that we might know God. The Holy Bible is like a window into the heart of God to behold Him and to see what God is really like. As a teacher and counselor of the Word of God, I found myself entering into a deeper and more intimate relationship with God when I made His Word personal to me. It was like a friend talking to a dear friend you love and respect.

> Taste and see that the LORD is good; blessed is the man who takes refuge in him. Fear the LORD, you his saints, for those who fear him lack nothing. The lions may grow weak and hungry, but those who seek the LORD lack no good thing.
>
> Psalms 34:8–10 NIV

We will never know what and who God really is unless we read and know His Word.

> In the beginning was the Word, and the Word was with God, and the Word was God. He was with God in the beginning. The Word is Jesus Christ written down for all to behold.
>
> John 1:1–2 NIV

It is God's best design, as stated in the Book of Timothy, that we teach each generation the Word of God. This is so that we can build each other up in faith especially during the arduous time of dealing with cancer.

> You then, my son, be strong in the grace that is in Christ Jesus. And the things you have heard me say in the presence of many witnesses entrust to reliable men who will also be qualified to teach others. Endure hardship with us like a good soldier of Christ Jesus.
>
> 2 Timothy 2:1–3 NIV

When we have a good foundation and rely on the truth of God's Word and His promises to us, we can go through this journey in peace weathering all the hard storms.

When we study what is real, we will recognize what is false. Why do I say that? Because having a firm foundation will help us immediately recognize any lies. As we know the Word of God, we will know Jesus:

> The Word became flesh and made his dwelling among us. We have seen his glory, the glory of the One and Only Jesus, who came from the Father, full of grace and truth.
>
> John 1:14 NIV

God wants us to have a personal knowledge of His faithfulness to us as we walk through the challenging circumstances of illness. As I talked to God in the middle of the night and all during the day, Jesus was real to me. It was not just an intellectual knowledge any longer; it was a true relationship with my God who I knew would never leave me nor forsake me. In moments when I was lonely or afraid, I held fast to the Word of God especially in Psalm 91.

> He who dwells in the shelter of the Most High will rest in the shadow of the Almighty. I will say of the LORD, "He is my refuge and my fortress, my God, in whom I trust."
>
> Psalms 91:1–2 NIV

As believing Christians, our lives might be the only Word of God someone else might ever see or know, as Paul states in the Book of Acts.

> You know that I have not hesitated to preach anything that would be helpful to you but have taught you publicly and from house to house. I have declared to both Jews and Greeks that they must turn to God in repentance and have faith in our Lord Jesus.
>
> Acts 20:20–21 NIV

Another comforting statement, for me knowing I could be facing possible death, was again from Paul. Paul declared he did not count his life dear except to testify of the hope in Jesus Christ.

> However, I consider my life worth nothing to me, if only I may finish the race and complete the task the Lord Jesus has given me—the task of testifying to the gospel of God's grace.
>
> Acts 20:24 NIV

God has entrusted us to share this wonderful gospel with all men. So even in the midst of tremendous suffering, our life can be a testimony of God's love, hope, and goodness. Thus, we see God's whole intention is that we would be transformed into His very nature through whatever hardship we face in this world.

> Do not conform any longer to the pattern of this world, but be transformed by the renewing of your mind. Then you will be able to test and approve what God's will is—his good, pleasing and perfect will.
>
> Romans 12:2 NIV

Chapter 7—Summary Of Transformed Into God's Character

Lesson Discussion:

Dr. Dees' statement, "Do you believe cancer can be a stairway to Heaven?"

Scripture Focus:

Philippians 3:10	That I may know Him. NIV
Psalm 63:1	Early will I seek Thee. NIV
Galatians 5:22	The Holy Spirit in our lives. NIV
Hebrews 10:38	The just shall live by faith. NIV

Doctor's Comments:

There is a patient who comes to mind immediately when I think how having cancer can affect one's life in a very positive way. He was operated on for throat cancer and tells his story openly in the F.R.I.E.N.D.S. Christian Cancer Care Support Group meetings.

Like most patients I meet on the first visit, this individual was fearful and eager to develop a "plan of attack" regarding his cancer treatment. Most patients who leave with such a plan, cease to be terrified with their diagnosis, and have new hope of resolution from their chemo regimen. But relying on the doctor is not the pathway to peace because *cancer management is more than medicine.*

This journey toward peace is best illustrated through this patient who relied on himself as a "self-made" man who believed in being totally "macho" and definitely independent. In his own words, "I was full of pride and ego. I will get through this by myself!"

Through his trial of cancer and his personal involvement with F.R.I.E.N.D.S. Christian Cancer Care, his whole life became more meaningful and much more peaceful. He then started getting up every day waiting for God's directions and not his own. You can definitely have cancer and experience peace and joy. However, the real answer to peace will not be found at the doctor's office, in the treatment, or in a bottle of medicine. F.R.I.E.N.D.S. Christian Cancer Care is for people looking for peace. We hope there will be many more that will join us in our journey of peace.

Topic Discussion Question:

How has your trial of cancer changed your understanding of true peace? Have you seen a difference in having intellectual knowledge of peace versus true spiritual understanding of peace?

Suggested Closing Prayer:

Thank you, Heavenly Father, that we are not conformed entirely to the knowledge and thinking of this temporary world, but we are being transformed daily by the renewing of our minds through your Holy Word, the Bible. Thank you, Lord, that you are the Prince of Peace and no matter what is going on in our lives we can have true peace in You. In Jesus' mighty name we pray. Amen.

Additional Follow-Up Scriptures:

2 Timothy 2:1	You then, my son, be strong in the grace that is in Christ Jesus. NIV
John 1: 1	Before anything else existed, there was Christ. NIV
John 1:14	The Word became flesh and made his dwelling among us. NIV
Acts 20:22–25	And now, compelled by the Spirit I am going. NIV
Romans 12: 2	Do not conform any longer to the pattern of this world, but be transformed by the renewing of your mind. NIV

Notes:

_____

_____

_____

_____

_____

_____

_____

_____

_____

_____

_____

_____

_____

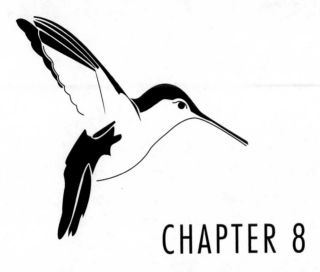

CHAPTER 8
Living with Passion and Purpose

Lesson Objective:

God Is Committed to Finishing the Good Work in Us

Scripture Focus:

2 Timothy 1:12	For the which cause I also suffer these things: nevertheless ... NIV
2 Timothy 1:14	That good thing which was committed unto thee keep by the Holy Ghost which dwelleth in us. NIV

Topic Discussion Question:

What is the greatest lesson you have learned during this trial, and how do you think you can help others now go through this challenge?

Suggested Prayer:

Heavenly Father, thank you that you are committed to us. Thank you that your commitment to us does not depend on how good we are, but it all depends on the shed blood of your Son, Jesus Christ. Thank you, Lord, you loved us so much that you gave up your Son that we would be free from sin and death. Thank you, Lord, that who the Son sets free is free indeed never to be returned to a yoke of bondage again. In Jesus' name. Amen.

Teaching:

> ...for I am Jehovah. The blood you have placed on the doorposts will be proof that you obey me, and when I see the blood I will pass over you and I will not destroy your firstborn children when I smite the land of Egypt. "You shall celebrate this event each year."
>
> Exodus 12:12–14 TLB

God was warning His people. He wanted them to make sure they applied the blood of the Lamb over the doorposts of their homes, so that the death angel would pass over. They did this so that the people inside the home where the blood had been applied would be kept safe.

These were believers in the one true God Jehovah, our Lord Jesus Christ. There were three types of people who could have been inside the homes: the fearful, the skeptical, or those filled with joy and hope knowing they were secure in God.

Isn't that just how it is for us, as believers, walking through disease and sickness that challenge our lives? The fearful and skeptical perhaps would be praying in earnest that God would spare their lives.

They probably felt they had disappointed God, or made God angry, and that is why they were sick in the first place. Then, there were those believers who were secure and filled with joy and were confident in the love God had for them.

God's deliverance is never based on our feelings or our fears. The deliverance God brings is based on the love, mercy, and shed blood of Jesus Christ at Calvary. In this portion of scripture, it was judgment day for Egypt.

> "On that same night I will pass through Egypt and strike down every firstborn—both men and animals—and I will bring judgment on all the gods of Egypt."
>
> Exodus 12:12 NIV

God was saying, "I will execute judgment over the powers of darkness that are trying to destroy your lives through curses and sickness of your past." God's deliverance was not based upon the behavior of each person: God's deliverance was based on His great mercy and love. These people were totally out of the will of God and backslidden from worshiping God. God was giving them another chance.

God has rescued me and delivered me out of past circumstances and present-day challenges, with overcoming cancer, to make a difference for Him. Our call at F.R.I.E.N.D.S. Christian Cancer Care, Inc. is to bring hope and comfort during the trial of cancer. God uses me even though I am far from being a perfect person.

> But God demonstrates his own love for us in this: While we were still sinners, Christ died for us. Since we have now been justified by his blood, how much more shall we be saved from God's wrath through him! For if, when we were God's enemies, we were reconciled to him through the death of his Son, how much more, having been reconciled, shall we be saved through his life! Not only is this so, but we also rejoice in God through our Lord Jesus Christ, through whom we have now received reconciliation.
>
> Romans 5:8–11 NIV

While we were all yet sinners, Christ died for us. Taking part in the Passover was so that they knew they were secure and being fully delivered based on the blood sacrifice. As believers in Christ, we can face each day with confidence and peace knowing we have absolute assurance in Christ Jesus to carry us through whatever we are facing in this journey called life.

The Old Testament Passover is a symbol of the blood of Jesus shed at Cavalry. Spiritually through prayer, we apply this blood over the doorposts of each of our hearts as believers in the Lord Jesus Christ.

The question we need to ask ourselves as believers is: Are we waiting with our attitudes and behavior with expectancy in the faithfulness of God, or are we waiting in fear? Are we waiting with the calm inner joy and peace that comes with confidence toward our God to be ever faithful and true, or are we in doubt, confusion, and dismay? The greater the trial in my life, the greater I try to stay pressed into God and His Word. It is what gives me passion and purpose to continue in this life with joy.

When we do not accept God's forgiveness and the price Jesus paid on Cavalry for our sins, we stay condemned, ashamed, and guilty. Many times, if we are not careful especially when challenged with an invasive disease, we can find ourselves being self-destructive out of anger or self-pity. Also, when we stay in condemnation and are ashamed, we can start to justify our sin and become more self-destructive through the sin in our lives.

The way to peace and deliverance is always repentance. This is my personal prayer, "God, I am wrong, and you are right. Please forgive me for any thought, word, or action that does not line up with your Word. Even though I do not feel forgiven sometimes, I thank you, Lord, that your Word says you forgive me and forget my transgressions." Most of us, especially if we are sick feel guilty. God wants us free from all sin and guilt.

God does not want our excuses or justified responses. God understands our need to prove Him right over and over again by following our own ways and not His Word.

However, God ultimately wants our hearts, and many times when we are quiet before Him, that is when we hear God's voice best.

During treatments, I was particularly weak and many times would call on God for His courage and grace. Because of my work ethic, I felt guilty not being able to work, but it was during this time I heard God's voice in my spirit and felt His presence the greatest. As I called on Him in my place of need, His love would overshadow every doubt, and peace would flood my heart.

> Draw me, we will run after thee: the king hath brought me into his chambers: we will be glad and rejoice in thee, we will remember thy love more than wine: the upright love thee.
>
> Song of Solomon 1:4 KJV

God runs to meet us when we turn our hearts toward Him. God understands when we are hurting. I really discovered this in my darkest moments of the cancer trial. Jesus sympathizes with our fears and weakness.

> For we do not have a high priest who is unable to sympathize with our weaknesses, but we have one who has been tempted in every way, just as we are—yet was without sin. Let us then approach the throne of grace with confidence, so that we may receive mercy and find grace to help us in our time of need.
>
> Hebrews 4:15–16 NIV

Repentance is a gift from God. Whatever we have on our hearts, we can bring it to God and be forgiven. God is able to subdue all things within us, even fear of pain and being alone. When we tell the Lord of our fears or shame, God comes and brings His presence, and a clearing comes from the refreshing presence of the Lord. God wants us to approach Him and come to Him in communication with no fear and no shame, only confidence.

> God says he will accept and acquit us—declare us "not guilty"—if we trust Jesus Christ to take away our sins. And we all can be saved in this same way, by coming to Christ, no matter who we are or what we have been like.
>
> Romans 3:21 TLB

When we turn to God, God comes running to meet us.

> Yes, all have sinned; all fall short of God's glorious ideal; 24 yet now God declares us "not guilty" of offending him if we trust in Jesus Christ, who in his kindness freely takes away our sins.
>
> Romans 3:23 TLB

As our spirits are clear from repentance, God can speak to us even when we are sick or challenged. God will and does breathe purpose and passion in our hearts once again, instead of despair. I am a perfect example of this. When I thought my life was totally over from having a purpose, God breathed passion in me to start F.R.I.E.N.D.S.

Christian Cancer Care, Inc. Out of a horrible disease, God brought something beautiful.

> ...to proclaim the year of the LORD's favor and the day of vengeance of our God, to comfort all who mourn, and provide for those who grieve in Zion—to bestow on them a crown of beauty instead of ashes, the oil of gladness instead of mourning, and a garment of praise instead of a spirit of despair. They will be called oaks of righteousness, a planting of the LORD for the display of his splendor.
>
> Isaiah 61:2–3 NIV

Chapter 8—Summary Of Living With Passion And Purpose With Cancer

Lesson Discussion:

We are more than a physical body, and God wants us to live with purpose and passion daily even when we are our weakest.

Scripture Focus:

James 1:6–8 — A double-minded man is unstable in all his ways. NIV

Hebrews 11:6 — God rewards those who diligently seek Him. NIV

Isaiah 54:1–17	No weapon forged against you will prevail. NIV
Acts 12:1–16	God is our source for everything. NIV
Daniel 9:2	I turned to the Lord with prayer and fasting. NIV

Doctor's Comments:

I hear patients say that their doctor is their hero. Certainly, that is a fantastic outcome of the complex doctor-patient relationship. I would like to write about a patient that is my hero and teaches me whenever I am lucky enough to spend some time with her. She was diagnosed with Lymphoma eight years ago and told she had three months to live. She tried chemotherapy, but as she said, God knew she could not tolerate the side effects. Instead she turned to prayer and the Bible.

Her cancer at one point hospitalized her and a lung biopsy proved that it had spread there, and she was short of breath. Another time her spleen was so enlarged it reached nearly down to her pelvis and she was very uncomfortable. She became anemic and fatigued. Each time she faced a physical crisis, she turned to God. He changed her language to one of healing, and charged her with comforting others. We all carry our "to do" list, but truthfully is there anything on that list that will bring us peace and everlasting life? I doubt it. She gets up every day and asks God for her direction and joyfully attends other's sorrow. She is my hero and she is a shining light in a world full of suffering. Her cancer is in remission.

Topic Discussion Question:

Is cancer my new identity? Or does God really want to reward me by giving me purpose and passion during this time?

Suggested Closing Prayer:

Lord, thank you that every time we come to you in faith You will carry us over, our faith pleases you; that Your name is Faithful and True and we can trust that our latter end will be far greater than our former end. We love You, Lord, and release our faith to do Your will. In Jesus' name. Amen.

Additional Follow-Up Scriptures:

1 John 5:13–15	This is the confidence we have in approaching God NIV
Romans 3:26–28	A man is justified by his faith NIV
Proverbs 6:27	Can a man bring fire into his lap without being burned? NIV
Jeremiah 29:11	For I know the plans I have for you NIV

Notes:

_____

_____

_____

_____

_____

_____

_____

_____

_____

_____

_____

_____

_____

_____

Rev. Lillian Elizabeth Barnhardt-Israel

_____

_____

_____

_____

_____

_____

_____

_____

_____

_____

_____

_____

_____

_____

CHAPTER 9

Faith Versus Doubt and Faulty Reasoning

Lesson Objective:

God wants us to move from the first stages of faith into complete trust in Him without any fear, doubt or faulty reasoning.

Scripture Focus:

Daniel 3:17–18

Our God whom we serve is able to deliver us. NIV

Topic Discussion Question:

While in the midst of the cancer struggle, what seems to cause you the most doubt?

Suggested Prayer:

Lord God, help us to believe you and your promises during this difficult challenge. Help us to keep our eyes on you and dwell in the presence of your Word that brings us peace, comfort, love, and hope. In Jesus' name. Amen

Teaching:

When we look at doubt, we need to look at the attitudes of our heart. When we are in the midst of violent attacks dealing with sickness the tendency is always to overreact in fear, doubt and faulty reasoning.

To stand in faith at this time, the first thing we have to believe is that our God is able to deliver us. God is not limited in His power or ability. God is all powerful. God's arm is not too short to rescue us. He is able to do all His Word says He can do.

Secondly, God is not a respecter of persons. We have to make a choice to believe not only is God able to deliver us, it is His divine will for each of us. There is a big difference in believing for someone else's healing, and believing in faith, that God will do it for you personally too. Many times, we think other people are more loved than us, or favored by God more than we are, or that God is mad at us.

If God does not deliver us out of the situation, He will go through the situation with us and give us grace to stand. This is my personal testimony of how I learned to be an overcomer through the heavy emotional tides of cancer.

> "But even if he does not, we want you to know, O king, that we will not serve your gods or worship the image of gold you have set up."
>
> Daniel 3:18 NIV

God only has the very best for each of us. Have you ever prayed for something and then were so grateful God chose to do it His way instead of your way? His way is always best for everyone involved.

Therefore, this is why it is so important when we are healed from cancer, and maybe someone else goes home to be with Jesus, we do not judge them wrongly. There has been wrong teaching that says, "If God does not answer your prayer, there is something wrong with your faith." This causes people condemnation. My own husband went home early to be with the Lord at fifty-six years old. It broke my heart, but I realize now God did the very best for all of us because his body was worn out, and he was ready to be with the Lord. The Bible says, we will know and understand things more, as we walk on with God.

> Then shall we know, if we follow on to know the LORD: his going forth is prepared as the morning; and he shall come unto us as the rain, as the latter and former rain unto the earth.
>
> Hosea 6:3 KJV

As we walk with God through life's journey, our faith will turn into complete trust. This means, that no matter what happens in our lives, we know God is trustworthy and will never leave us nor forsake us.

> Therefore we will not fear, though the earth give way and the mountains fall into the heart of the sea, though its waters roar and foam and the mountains quake with their surging.
>
> Psalms 46:2–3 NIV

The place of trust in God is greater than faith. Faith is built on experience. Trust says that when the tests come, I know the person of God, and no matter what my circumstances look like or what I am facing, I can truthfully say, "Lord, I trust you. I trust your timing, Lord, and that you know what is best for me." When we are able to acknowledge this truth, we move from faith to a place of complete trust.

It may be a year or so before we can look back and say, "Oh Lord, you knew exactly what was best for me and what you were doing in my life. Lord, you always know what is best for everyone involved in each situation." When this happens in our lives, doubt will have to leave and faith will replace all fear.

Faulty reasoning will keep us from coming into the full plan of God, and faulty reasoning and doubt will destroy our faith. The following Bible verse best exemplifies my statement.

When they had crossed, Elijah said to Elisha, "Tell me, what can I do for you before I am taken from you?" "Let me inherit a double portion of *your spirit*," Elisha replied. "You have asked a difficult thing," Elijah said, "yet if you see me when I am taken from you, it will be yours—otherwise not."

As they were walking along and talking together, suddenly a chariot of fire and horses of fire appeared and separated the two of them, and Elijah went up to heaven in a whirlwind. Elisha saw this and cried out, "My father! My father! The chariots and horsemen of Israel!" And Elisha saw him no more.

Then he took hold of his own clothes and tore them apart. He picked up the cloak that had fallen from Elijah and went back and stood on the bank of the Jordan. Then he took the cloak that had fallen from him and struck the water with it. "Where now is the LORD, the God of Elijah?" he asked. When he struck the water, it divided to the right and to the left, and he crossed over. The company of the prophets from Jericho, who were watching, said, "The spirit of Elijah is resting on Elisha." And they went to meet him and bowed to the ground before him.

2 Kings 2:9–15 NIV

Elisha received the double-portion anointing of the presence of God in his life, because Elisha never took his eyes off Elijah, even when all around him was in total chaos. This has always been one of my favorite Bible stories of diligence and commitment. Even when we are not perfect or particularly gifted, we can be faithful and diligent in our faith toward God, and God will count it unto us as righteousness and reward us.

There were moments of time during my treatment, I felt I could not go another step and wanted to quit. But, God would strengthen my heart to keep my eyes fixed on Him and not my circumstances, and through His grace I was able to continue.

When we take our eyes off of Jesus and His faithfulness in our lives, our hearts want to sink just like the story of Peter in the Book of Matthew. We can start off being full of strength and resolve, but as time goes on and we are surrounded by tumultuous circumstances, our hearts want to sink.

> During the fourth watch of the night Jesus went out to them, walking on the lake. When the disciples saw him walking on the lake, they were terrified. "It's a ghost," they said, and cried out in fear. But Jesus immediately said to them: "Take courage! It is I. Don't be afraid." "Lord, if it's you," Peter replied, "tell me to come to you on the water." "Come," he said. Then Peter got down out of the boat, walked on the water and came toward Jesus. But when he saw the wind, he was afraid and, beginning to sink, cried out, "Lord, save me!" Immediately Jesus reached out His hand and caught him. "You of little faith," he said, "why did you doubt?"
>
> Matthew 14:25–31 NIV

Whenever my heart is sinking and the voices of my circumstances scream at me, I recount the faithfulness of God over my life. God has been faithful even when I was not, and I can trust Him to take me through whatever trial I am facing. The Word of God read and repeated was the only thing that kept me from faulty reasoning so many times. We do not have all the details of our future and understand all that God is doing behind the scenes, but God promises us in His Word, He will never allow more than we can handle.

When the disciples saw Jesus crucified, their dreams were dashed and their hearts were broken. They began to think their lives were over at the loss of Jesus through the crucifixion. Jesus was gone, and they began to judge their circumstances through faulty reasoning rather than what was true.

> And their words seemed to them as idle tales, and they believed them not. Peter, however, got up and ran to the tomb. Bending over, he saw the strips of linen lying by themselves, and he went away, wondering to himself what had happened. Now that same day, two of them were going to a village called Emmaus, about seven miles from Jerusalem. They were talking with each other about everything that had happened.
>
> Luke 24:11–14 NIV

When we are in the midst of hard trials, especially when weak with sickness or when someone we love is very sick, we start to judge our circumstances and we forget the faithfulness of God. We get in unbelief, and it is easy to have faulty reasoning smothered in doubt.

> And it came to pass, that, while they communed together and reasoned, Jesus himself drew near, and went with them. But their eyes were holden that they should not know him. And he said unto them, What manner of communications are these that ye have one to another, as ye walk, and are sad?
>
> Luke 24:15–17 KJV

When we are in the pain and anguish of our cancer trial, it is not easy to keep our feelings from overtaking us and controlling us rather than what we know is true in the Word of God. The disciples began to live by their feelings, and they spoke about all the horrible things that had happened regarding Jesus. Although, the crucifixion was God's plan to save humanity, in the disciples' reasoning their loss of Jesus told them a total failure had occurred. They believed this through faulty reasoning, because Jesus was no longer with them. God's reasoning said total victory had been wrought for them, but they did not recognize the truth.

> He said to them, "How foolish you are, and how slow of heart to believe all that the prophets have spoken! Did not the Christ have to suffer these things and then enter his glory?" And beginning with Moses and all the Prophets, he explained to them what was said in all the Scriptures concerning himself. As they approached the village to

which they were *going*, Jesus acted as if he were going farther. But they urged him strongly, "Stay with us, for it is nearly evening; the day is almost over." So he went in to stay with them. When he was at the table with them, he took bread, gave thanks, broke it and began to give it to them. Then their eyes were opened and they recognized him, and he disappeared from their sight. They asked each other, "Were not our hearts burning within us while he talked with us on the road and opened the Scriptures to us?" They got up and returned at once to Jerusalem. There they found the Eleven and those with them, assembled together and saying, "It is true! The Lord has risen and has appeared to Simon." Then the two told what had happened on the way, and how Jesus was recognized by them when he broke the bread.

Luke 24:25–35 NIV

The truth was not in their reasoning or their feelings. The truth was in the fact that the Lord Jesus Christ had risen. Because He lives, we live. This is the truth, this is our evidence and this is our promise that cancer may roar at us, but as we trust God we will walk in faith and not faulty reasoning and doubt.

Then Jesus told him, "Because you have seen me, you have believed; blessed are those who have not seen and yet have believed."

John 20:29 NIV

Chapter 9—Summary Of Faith Versus Doubt And Faulty Reasoning

Lesson Discussion:

How faulty reasoning and doubt can cause us great physical stress as well as emotional stress.

Scripture Focus:

1 Peter 1:3	God has given us a new hope NIV
Daniel 3:17	God is able NIV
Matthew 14:25–31	You of little faith NIV
Luke 24:11–15	Do not be sad NIV

Doctor's Comments:

There are people who do not want to submit to medical treatment because of doubt and faulty reasoning. But it is important to understand life experiences that have found you to want to be in control of your treatment and destiny. Certainly there is not enough known about effects of diet. The best evidence supports nutritious diet. Beyond this, our research is lacking. I had a patient with metastatic cancer with no medical cure who my nurses and I treated for nearly ten years.

When she passed away, we knew little about this person, and no one seemed to know anyone who knew her. Word was left that she wanted me to speak at her funeral, which under the circumstances I felt was unusual. I thought it would be helpful if I would speak for her. I found out this person was diagnosed several years ago. She had given interviews and even helped other families during this time.

The cancer reoccurred. No one knew what was going on. She did not take any medicine or treatments. She tried other alternative regimens. Finally she decided, with difficulty, to do some treatments. She did not continue. A statement during the funeral was made regarding "how copacetic all her relationships were but there were obstacles from the past." It appeared she allowed cancer to destroy her because she had no trust, and she never felt valuable enough because of the abuse and control she had suffered in her past.

Topic Discussion Question:

Considering doubt and faulty reasoning, can you pinpoint a time when this affected your choices with medical treatment or relationships?

Suggested Closing Prayer:

Heavenly Father, help us to remember that when we feel as we have been thrown into a fiery trial, Your promises are 'yes' and 'amen' to all who believe. You, our God, whom we serve, are able to deliver us from the burning fiery furnace, and you will deliver us out of the enemy's hand. We believe you can, you are able and you will. But no matter what happens or what the circumstances are, we choose to believe and trust in You! In Jesus' mighty name. Amen."

Additional Follow-Up Scriptures:

2 Kings 2:9–30   Elijah said to Elisha, "Keep
your eyes fixed on me." NIV

Notes:

_____

_____

_____

_____

_____

_____

_____

_____

_____

_____

_____

CHAPTER 10

Acceptance

Lesson Objective:

We can be accepting because we know we are accepted in the beloved Jesus Christ.

Scripture Focus:

Ephesians 1:6	To the praise and glory of His grace, wherein he hath made us accepted in the beloved. NIV
Psalms 16:8–12	God is at my right hand and I shall not be moved. NIV

Topic Discussion Question:

How have you been challenged in feeling loved and accepted?

Suggested Prayer:

Lord, thank you that whatever we are facing today, you are bigger than any circumstance and that you are in control of our lives. Therefore, we do not have to be moved off of a place of complete faith in You because You have the very highest and best for us with the most excellent end. In Jesus' name. Amen

Teaching:

Understanding acceptance in God is a powerful force in our lives to be able to accept and weather the storms.

> To the praise and glory of His grace, wherein He hath made us accepted in the beloved.
>
> Ephesians 1:6 KJV

The word *acceptance*, according to Daniel Webster's II Collegiate Dictionary, means to get in agreement, approval, or be in agreement with another person.

When diagnosed with cancer, or when someone we love is diagnosed with cancer, it is a shock. Immediately our minds race with this devastating news, and how it will affect our lives. The last thing that comes to our mind is acceptance, but I have learned that the minute I am aware of painful news out of my control, I have to surrender the situation to God. God assures us that He will take all things in our lives and work them for our good, if we make a decision to let Him. In the middle of the night, during the hardest time of my treatments, I was alone. It was then that this promise became a true reality.

> And we know that all things work together for good to them that love God, to them who are the called according to his purpose.
>
> Romans 8:28 KJV

God had taken many bad circumstances in my life and turned them into something good. However, at the time, I could not see how God was going to use this trial and turn it for good that night. But, He did, and F.R.I.E.N.D.S. Christian Cancer Care, Inc. was born.

Back in 2006, Dr. Dees said, "Cancer patients do not have a prayer. Liz, would you please write a prayer for cancer patients?" The prayer was written in those early morning hours with God when I thought my life was over, and at the same time, God birthed the plan for F.R.I.E.N.D.S. As I surrendered my heart by making a choice to ask God to take this situation and turn it for good, God did turn it for good and birthed in my heart the "Prayer of a Doctor and a Patient."

In our lives, many times, we reason about things at a given time in our experience and reasoning tells us one thing, when the truth is actually something quite different. God wants us to trust Him completely by accepting His Word and being in agreement with Him, and what His promises declare, no matter what events are affecting our lives.

Joseph was a wonderful example of acceptance in the face of hardship.

> But Joseph said to them, "Don't be afraid. Am I in the place of God? You intended to harm me, but God intended it for good to accomplish what is now being done, the saving of many lives. So then, don't be afraid."
>
> Genesis 50:19–21 NIV

When God allows me to go through a trial now, my attitude toward the challenge has been changed greatly. I have come to realize God has entrusted me, with the trials of life, so that I may grow in a personal knowledge of Him and His faithfulness. I can accept whatever life throws my way because I know God totally accepts me. This gives me confidence toward God and the grace to stand.

Wherein, He has made us accepted in the beloved means total acceptance in God, with total pardon for every sin and receiving total favor by God. God's acceptance is the unconditional love of God in our lives.

> Nor height, nor depth, nor any other creature, shall be able to separate us from the love of God, which is in Christ Jesus our Lord.
>
> Romans 8:39 KJV

Knowing we are accepted makes the difference in good marriages, stable children and all our relationships. When we are unsure of our acceptance by someone, we are insecure and reluctant to communicate with trust. Acceptance is also key in good business management. Unless people feel valuable, they will never perform to their best potential.

As we mature as Christians, it is vital for us to know our acceptance in God's unconditional love. It will enable us to endure in faith through our trials and heartbreak of cancer and all its challenges. Having a knowledge of our acceptance, will allow us to be confident without a doubt that God is trustworthy and faithful.

God wants us established in His love forever. All through my diagnosis, surgeries, treatments, and all that followed, God would speak to my spirit, "Liz, never forget how much I love you. My love never quits. My mercies are new every morning."

> The Lord appeared from of old to me [Israel], say-
> ing, Yes, I have loved you with an everlasting love;
> therefore with loving-kindness have I drawn you
> and continued My faithfulness to you.
>
> Jeremiah 31:3 AMP

God loves us with an everlasting love. His love never comes to an end and His love knows no boundaries. It is not what God does, but who He is as the person of God.

We have to remember this when we are suffering pain and hardship or someone we love is, that is why the Word of God was given to us.

> For this reason I kneel before the Father, from whom
> his whole family in heaven and on earth derives its
> name. I pray that out of his glorious riches he may
> strengthen you with power through his Spirit in

your inner being, so that Christ may dwell in your hearts through faith. And I pray that you, being rooted and established in love, may have power, together with all the saints, to grasp how wide and long and high and deep is the love of Christ, and to know this love that surpasses knowledge—that you may be filled to the measure of all the fullness of God. Now to him who is able to do immeasurably more than all we ask or imagine, according to his power that is at work within us, to him be glory in the church and in Christ Jesus throughout all generations, forever and ever! Amen.

Ephesians 3:14–21 NIV

Paul prayed for the church at Ephesus that they would come to fully know how much God loved them. God wants us all to be secure in His love for us because God knew many of our problems would arise out of being insecure and not understanding how much He loves us.

As long as we are on this earth, we will be challenged in our physical bodies with aging and staying healthy until it is our time to go home to be with the Lord. We were born in the Lord's heart before the beginning of time. It is out of God's heart we came, and it will be to the Lord's heart we will return to spend all eternity in fellowship with Him. Therefore, God wants us to be secure in our acceptance by Him as long as we are on this earth.

"Before I formed you in the womb I knew you, before you were born I set you apart; I appointed you as a prophet to the nations."

Jeremiah 1:5 AMP

"For I know the plans I have for you," declares the LORD, "plans to prosper you and not to harm you, plans to give you hope and a future. Then you will call upon me and come and pray to me, and I will listen to you. You will seek me and find me when you seek me with all your heart."

Jeremiah 29:11–13 NIV

Acceptance in God is simply agreeing with His Word, and what He says about us and to us!

Chapter 10—Summary Of Acceptance

Lesson Discussion:

Finding out how our Lord can take very bitter circumstances and make them turn to something sweet.

Scripture Focus:

Genesis 50:19	God meant it for good NIV
Ephesians 1:6	God has made us accepted. NIV
Ephesians 2:7	God expressed His kindness in Jesus. NIV
Psalms 16:8–12	God is at my right hand—I shall not be moved! NIV

Doctor's Comments:

I had a female patient who had received a very severe shock medically from another medical professional. Personally, I believe our life is more than a physical body.

She, the patient, was diagnosed with acute Myeloid Leukemia. Very few adults walk away from this disease. I met her in a small, dimly lit, dingy hospital room, and as I gazed out the window, all I could see was a long row of telephone poles over barren soil. She pointed out to me that these were reminders of crosses signifying God's grace and love.

Her light spirit brightened up my visits to her room for over four months where she withstood induction chemo-therapy and four additional hospital readmissions for blood transfusions. She celebrated her birthday in the hospital, and all the nurses were drawn to her by her great spirit. Even today, five years from the original diagnosis, she lights up our F.R.I.E.N.D.S. Christian Cancer Care support group!

Topic Discussion Question:

How has knowing you are accepted and loved by God, help you at this time?

Suggested Closing Prayer:

Heavenly Father, we thank you that it is Your desire for each of us to be established in Your love forever. Thank you, Lord, that you have loved us with an everlasting love and drawn us with your loving kindness. God, thank you for Your continued faithfulness toward us today and every day! In Jesus' name. Amen.

Additional Follow-Up Scriptures:

Jeremiah 31:3 … I have drawn you with loving-kindness. NIV

Ephesians 3:14 For this reason I kneel before the Father. NIV

Notes:

_____

_____

_____

_____

_____

_____

_____

_____

Rev. Lillian Elizabeth Barnhardt-Israel

CHAPTER 11

Redemption

Lesson Objective:

When we are diagnosed, or when someone we love is diagnosed with cancer, we need to know we are forgiven and redeemed by our Lord, Jesus Christ.

Scripture Focus:

Ephesians 2:13   We need to know we are forgiven. NIV

Romans 3:24   Being justified freely by His grace in Christ Jesus. NIV

Topic Discussion Question:

Why do I have a hard time believing I am truly forgiven?

Suggested Prayer:

Lord Jesus, it is easy to forget when we are overwhelmed that You are committed to us forever. Please help us remember You have redeemed us, rescued us and saved us eternally. Thank You Lord that our redemption does not depend on our faithfulness, but the faithfulness of our almighty God! In Jesus' name. Amen

Teaching:

A simple explanation of the word redeemed means to be rescued or liberated from sin, as stated in the Daniel Webster's II Collegiate Dictionary. This is the true ministry of our Lord Jesus Christ. As our Savior, He came to set us free daily from the sin and bondage that would destroy our lives. God does not want us confused about our eternal security in Him. Jesus explains this as being set free. Facing terminal illness demands our dependence and knowledge of Him.

> How sayest thou, Ye shall be made free ? 34 Jesus answered them, Verily, verily, I say unto you, Whosoever committeth sin is the servant of sin. 35 And the servant abideth not in the house for ever: but the Son abideth ever. 36 If the Son therefore shall make you free , ye shall be free indeed.
>
> John 8:33 KJV

God wants us secure in His love, forgiveness, and peace. God does not want us insecure. God reminds us several times throughout the scriptures in the Old and New Testament that He is always with us.

> "Be strong and courageous. Do not be afraid or terrified because of them, for the LORD your God goes with you; he will never leave you nor forsake you."
>
> Deuteronomy 31:6 NIV

> And we know that Christ, God's Son, has come to help us understand and find the true God. And now we are in God because we are in Jesus Christ his Son, who is the only true God; and he is eternal Life.
>
> 1 John 5:20 TLB

It is important to understand that God's glory, His presence and character, is working in us even when we are suffering with cancer or terminal illness.

> The Spirit himself testifies with our spirit that we are God's children. Now if we are children, then we are heirs—heirs of God and co-heirs with Christ, if indeed we share in his sufferings in order that we may also share in his glory. I consider that our present sufferings are not worth comparing with the glory that will be revealed in us.
>
> Romans 8:16–18 NIV

Everyone will go through times of trial and challenge, but as believers in Christ, we are being changed from strength to strength and glory to glory as God transforms us by His redeeming love.

Even in our suffering, we can share the love and forgiveness of God because we are redeemed and confident God loves us. We can be at total peace knowing we are forgiven when we have repented. Then we are ready for heaven, if the Lord decides our healing will be on heaven's side of eternity.

> "Where, O death, is your victory? Where, O death, is your sting ?" The sting of death is sin, and the power of sin is the law. But thanks be to God! He gives us the victory through our Lord Jesus Christ.
> 1 Corinthians 15:55–57 NIV

The more we understand our need for a savior and a redeemer, the more liberty we have to call out to Him in times of need. This became particularly important as I faced being affected by cancer in so many different ways. First I was a caregiver, then a patient, and now I am involved medically and professionally with thousands affected by cancer. Reminding myself that when God promises to redeem me, He is saying to me I have come to liberate you and rescue you from your present state. It then makes it easier for me to roll the cares of what I face daily over onto His shoulders as my Redeemer.

> Jesus answered him, "Simon, I have something to tell you." "Tell me, teacher," he said. "Two men owed money to a certain moneylender. One owed him five hundred denarii, and the other fifty. Neither of them had the money to pay him back,

so he canceled the debts of both. Now which of them will love him more?" Simon replied, "I suppose the one who had the bigger debt canceled." "You have judged correctly," Jesus said.

Luke 7:40–43 NIV

During illness, we can rest in the redemption of Christ and His great love for us. We are grateful and realize the price He paid for our forgiveness. We do not have to fear because Jesus paid the ultimate price for our forgiveness. This always brought me comfort knowing God's grace would take me through any challenge I was facing.

When I was tempted to be in self-pity because I was alone much of the time, I would recount all the times God had saved me and rescued me in situations, even when I wasn't praying or walking with Him. Jesus was faithful even when I was not! Jesus describes in the Book of Luke, the heart of one who is truly grateful for the forgiveness of sin.

Then he turned toward the woman and said to Simon, "Do you see this woman? I came into your house. You did not give me any water for my feet, but she wet my feet with her tears and wiped them with her hair. You did not give me a kiss, but this woman, from the time I entered, has not stopped kissing my feet. You did not put oil on my head, but she has poured perfume on my feet. Therefore, I tell you, her many sins have been forgiven—for she loved much. But he who has been forgiven little loves little." Then Jesus said to her, "Your sins are forgiven."

Luke 7:44–48 NIV

The more we understand the great gift of redemption and that Jesus paid a price for us we could not pay, we will be able to remind ourselves in difficult times to be grateful. When we are sincerely grateful, there is a supernatural peace that fills our hearts because we know God hears us and is with us.

> "I will save you from the hands of the wicked and redeem you from the grasp of the cruel."
>
> Jeremiah 15:21 NIV

> I waited patiently for the LORD; he turned to me and heard my cry. He lifted me out of the slimy pit, out of the mud and mire; he set my feet on a rock and gave me a firm place to stand. He put a new song in my mouth, a hymn praise to our God. Many will see and fear and put their trust in the LORD. Blessed is the man who makes the LORD his trust.
>
> Psalms 40:1–4 NIV

Chapter 11—Summary Of Redemption

Lesson Discussion:

We need to know we are forgiven and loved in Jesus. How does our understanding of redemption affect us?

Scripture Focus:

Ephesians 2:13

We need to know who we are in Christ. NIV

Romans 3:24	We are justified by grace. NIV
1 Peter 1:2	To have freedom from stress and fear. NIV
Deuteronomy 31:6	God will never leave us nor forsake us. NIV
Psalms 84:5	Blessed are those whose trust is in God. NIV

Doctor's Comments:

I met with a patient who had a lung mass with lung cancer. He said, "I deserve to die." As the mass was small, he had a chance for a cure. He did not want to be referred for surgery. Curiously, I tried to get to know him better and found out he had fought in WWII for the Germans. He described his battlefield experience on the Russian front. Afterwards, he and his wife immigrated to America. This couple was shunned at work and socially. One day they got the nerve to ask the question, "Why?" This couple was told of the atrocities they had a part in and were shocked, but later had to accept what their countrymen had done.

This man did not feel he deserved to live because of the guilt and so he rejected all treatment. He had absolutely no value for his life and refused to acknowledge his need to develop a spiritual life and be forgiven. His cancer did progress, and he spent his final journey in guilt and shame.

Topic Discussion Question:

What is the biggest area of challenge you are facing in order for you to be at peace and rest in your own life? Do you need to forgive someone, yourself or God?

Suggested Closing Prayer:

Heavenly Father, thank You that Your Word declares, "Blessed is the man whose transgressions are forgiven and whose sins are covered. Blessed is the man whose sin the Lord does not count against him and in whose spirit there is no deceit." Lord God, thank You that You love us so much and gave us a way through Your holy Son, Jesus, to be forgiven of all of our sins. You said, "Whoever calls on the name of the Lord shall be saved from their sin." We call on You today, Lord. We acknowledge Jesus is the Son of God who died for us to be free. We receive Your forgiveness today in Jesus' mighty name! Amen.

Additional Follow-Up Scriptures:

Psalms 32:1–2	Blessed is he whose transgressions are forgiven, whose sins are covered. NIV
Luke 7:40–48	Jesus said, who loves the most…? NIV
Psalms 40:1–4	I waited patiently for the LORD; he turned to me and heard my cry. NIV

Jeremiah 15:21

"I will save you from the hands of the wicked and redeem you from the grasp of the cruel." NIV

Notes:

_____

_____

_____

_____

_____

_____

_____

_____

_____

_____

_____

Rev. Lillian Elizabeth Barnhardt-Israel

CHAPTER 12

There Is a Rest and Hope
for the People of God

Lesson Objective:

There is abundant rest and provision for the people of God

Scripture Focus:

Jeremiah 29:11

"For I know the plans I have for you," declares the Lord, "plans to prosper you and not to harm you, plans to give you hope and a future." NIV

Psalms 91:1	He who dwells in the shelter of the Most High *will rest* in the shadow (in the presence) of the Almighty. NIV

Topic Discussion Question:

What is the biggest area of challenge for you to be in hope and enter into a rest?

Suggested Prayer:

Lord God, we thank you that you are our shield from the storms of life. Heavenly Father, we thank you that you came that we would have life on this earth and have it to the fullest no matter what the circumstances. May your unfailing love rest upon us, even as we put our hope and faith in you. In Jesus' name. Amen.

Teaching:

God promises us there is a rest in His presence. It has become evident to me that rest and hope go hand in hand. As I am able to rest in God, my hope is also established.

> May your unfailing love rest upon us, O LORD, even as we put our hope in you.
>
> Psalms 33:22 NIV

Why is it necessary to know we need to hope and rest in God? Because the joy of the Lord is our strength, and we especially need all our strength to fight illness. It is imperative we understand and accept that there is a real enemy after our soul and our physical well being. This will help us in the fight against oppression, depression and fear that wants to overwhelm us at times of physical weakness and illness.

> The thief comes only to steal and kill and destroy; [but Jesus said,] I have come that they may have life, and have it to the full. I am the good shepherd. The good shepherd lays down his life for the sheep.
>
> John 10:10–11 NIV

At times when our hearts are faint or weak, it is the confidence toward God that bring us our rest.

> Who will be my shield? I would have died unless the Lord had helped me. I cried out, "I'm slipping, Lord!" and he was kind and saved me. Lord, when doubts fill my mind, when my heart is in turmoil, quiet me and give me renewed hope and cheer.
>
> Psalms 94:16–19 TLB

As we pour out our hearts to God in trust, our strength is renewed.

> For thus said the Lord God, the Holy One of Israel: In returning [to Me] and resting [in Me] you shall be saved; in quietness and in [trusting] confidence shall be your strength.
>
> Isaiah 30:15 AMP

When circumstances do not make sense, we can trust the heart of God, hope in Him, and find rest and comfort.

> Find rest, O my soul, in God alone; my hope comes from him. He alone is my rock and my salvation; he is my fortress, I will not be shaken. My salvation and my honor depend on God; he is my mighty rock, my refuge. Trust in him at all times, O people; pour out your hearts to him, for God is our refuge.
>
> Psalms 62:5–8 NIV

God wants us to bring all our burdens and heaviness to Him. We were not meant to be burden bearers, and if we insist on trying to carry our cares alone, we will find it will wear us down.

> Come to me and I will give you rest—all of you who work so hard beneath a heavy yoke. Wear my yoke—for it fits perfectly—and let me teach you; for I am gentle and humble, and you shall find rest for your souls; for I give you only light burdens.
>
> Matthew 11:28–29 NIV

God's yoke in the Greek means His will for our lives. His will for our lives brings us peace. Even in the midst of illness, we can depend on our God to rescue and deliver us through His grace and peace.

David with all his mistakes was a man after God's heart. When the yoke of life got too hard and too much, David cried out to the Lord.

Lord, hear my prayer! Listen to my plea! Don't turn away from me in this time of my distress. Bend down your ear and give me speedy answers, for my days disappear like smoke. My health is broken, and my heart is sick; it is trampled like grass and is withered. I lie awake, lonely as a solitary sparrow on the roof. My enemies taunt me day after day and curse at me. I eat ashes instead of bread. My tears run down into my drink because of your anger against me, because of your wrath. For you have rejected me and thrown me out. My life is passing swiftly as the evening shadows. I am withering like grass.

Psalms 102:1–3, 7–11 TLB

David's plea in the above-referenced scripture, is what we call today modern day depression, anxiety, and hopelessness. This happens especially when we are sick with cancer, because we often feel our future is uncertain, our goals are interrupted, and our hearts are broken with the sorrow of the situation. Fear wants to set in and it is followed by just plain weariness. Just as David cried out to God, I found I had to do this also during this season in my life. As I acknowledged God in all my ways, then my heart would be lifted up in hope toward God and His faithfulness.

He will listen to the prayers of the destitute, for he is never too busy to heed their requests.

Psalms 102:17 TLB

David's experience with God taught him that even though his heart could be breaking over his circumstances, he learned that weeping endures for the night but joy would come in the morning.

> …weeping may endure for a night, but joy cometh in the morning.
>
> Psalms 30:5 KJV

This scripture definitely became a reality for me when God brought a very special cancer patient into my life. His name was Jon. I met Jon at one of my lowest points while struggling through my remaining radiation treatments. It had already been close to nine months of surgeries, chemo and then radiation for me. The day I met Jon, I had made up my mind on the radiation table that I was sick and tired of going through this process. I had already quit in my heart, I just needed to let Dr. Dees be informed. As I walked out of the radiation treatment room into the lobby, there sat this precious young man with his mother.

As I had become accustomed to doing, I walked over and asked how they were, and if I could help them in any way. Jon was losing his hair, had a chemotherapy bag around his neck and was pale with physical weakness. As he looked up at me with huge brown eyes that were quietly desperate, he stated, "If I could only meet the lady who wrote this brochure, it would mean everything to me and my mother. It is bringing me such comfort." Of course as God would have it, the lady he wanted to meet was me. The brochure he was holding was the one Dr. Dees had asked me to write for F.R.I.E.N.D.S. Christian Cancer

Care. From that moment on, I chose to quit focusing on my own problems and gave my whole heart to helping others in the horrendous battle of cancer. I introduced myself, and the three of us became close friends.

Several times, I met with Jon's mother to comfort her regarding her son. During that time, I also met with Jon. One particular time, they called me to the hospital and asked me to pray for Jon. I asked very specifically what his request was. Jon asked me to pray that he could go home, that his nausea would subside, and that the pain would stop. Jon was ready to go on to be with our Lord Jesus. Jon was ready for his promotion into wholeness, but he asked specifically to be at home and not in the hospital.

It was a great privilege for me to be able to pray the prayer of faith for Jon with Jon and his mother. I asked specifically that God would grant Jon's requests. God did. My prayer was that Jon would be able to leave the hospital, be free of nausea and pain, and God would make his transition into eternity an easy one with joy.

From the day I met Jon, because of pain, Jon had not ever been able to smile. However, God did a miracle on behalf of this young man. Jon was able to leave the hospital and go home the next morning. At that particular time, it had been raining for several weeks in Florida, and the skies stayed dark and grey. However, Jon was able to rest in his own room and watch the rain through his bedroom window. That same night, Jon's mother called me and was very shaken. I went to her immediately. We met in the parking lot of the drug store she needed to go to for Jon's prescription. As I held her and prayed for her, she cried and released the pain of her grief and sorrow. God met her there, and she was able to return to Jon in peace and faith.

The following morning was Sunday, and I was in the first service at my church when I received a phone call from Jon's mother. She told me that he had asked her for a milkshake. She recalled to me that she was worried it was going to make him sick, but she decided to grant his request anyway. Jon's mother had lost her husband and Jon's father to cancer the year before, but her faith in God was still strong.

She went on to tell me in this phone conversation that Jon was able to drink the milkshake and keep it down. She also went on to say that for the first time in many months she saw Jon smile as he looked out the window, where it was still raining. She said he asked her if she could see the beautiful light coming through the window. This we both knew, at that moment, was the light of God flooding Jon's heart. We also both knew Jon was experiencing the glory of the Lord. His mother then told me with great emotion, Jon kept asking her if she could see the brilliant sunlight. "Do you see it mama-do you see it? Even though it was still raining Jon experienced the light of God filling his room. Lastly, she was able to tell me, at that moment Jon started laughing and she watched as he crossed over into eternity looking into the face of Jesus!

In the same way, we can see and understand only a little about God now, as if we were peering at his reflection in a poor mirror; but someday we are going to see him in his completeness, face to face.

Now all that I know is hazy and blurred, but then
I will see everything clearly, just as clearly as God
sees into my heart right now.

1 Corinthians 13:12 TLB

Jon received the ultimate and total healing. Jon received the ultimate promotion of rest, peace, and joy on a Sunday morning when his room was flooded with the light of Christ Jesus. Some of us are healed on this side of eternity, and some are healed on the other side of eternity. But God promises wholeness and healing to us all. As a cancer overcomer, I have decided that I want my life to count no matter how many days I have left on this earth. It is my desire, that all my remaining days be filled with faith, purpose, and passion.

He who dwells in the shelter of the Most High
will rest in the shadow of the Almighty. I will say
of the LORD, "He is my refuge and my fortress, my
God, in whom I trust."

Psalms 91:1–2 NIV

Chapter 12 Summary—Of There Is A Rest And Hope For The People Of God

Lesson Discussion:

Sometimes God takes us off-road in this journey called life.

Scripture Focus:

Jereremiah 29:11	God has plans to prosper us. NIV
Psalms 91:1	Rest in the shelter of the almighty. NIV
John 10:10	Jesus came that we would have life. NIV
Psalms 94:16	The Lord helped me. NIV
Isaiah 30:15	In quietness and confidence shall be my strength. NIV

Doctor's Comments:

With the diagnosis of cancer, you feel your future is changed forever, and you are not sure what your future holds. This is when many patients begin to assess their spiritual well-being and relationship with God.

I had a patient who knew early on he had advanced cancer. He was thirty-two years old. He assessed his life and realized that he had fallen short of pursuing spiritual well-being and peace. He was totally open to God's presence now.

He latched on to a prayer Rev. Lillian Elizabeth Barnhardt-Israel had written for our F.R.I.E.N.D.S. Christian Cancer Care Group. As he sat in the waiting room with his mother, they prayed he would meet Elizabeth, and they did. Liz emerged from treatment herself that day quite worn out and discouraged, but she had written the "Prayer of a Doctor and a Patient" from a request I made the first week I met her, and she knew she couldn't give up now.

I felt cancer patients didn't have a prayer, and I asked Liz to write a prayer so that I could put in my office: thus F.R.I.E.N.D.S. was born. Liz had been diagnosed with Stage 3C Breast Cancer and had endured surgery, chemotherapy, and radiation treatment. She often stated, "Whatever the outcome, I want to bring honor to God through this cancer journey. Then it will all be worth it!"

It was not by chance, we believe, God had Liz meet Jon and his mother that same afternoon they were praying in the waiting room of the cancer center. Later, Liz said, "Through that meeting, God sealed in my heart what He had trusted me to do, and that was to take F.R.I.E.N.D.S. and God's hope to as many as I could reach in cancer centers around the world."

After reading the prayer Liz had written, Jon realized there was more to life than inevitable death. He pursued real answers and eternal life with a real passion. It became our privilege to watch as Jon and his mother called on the Lord throughout the rest of his life's journey.

Rev. Lillian Elizabeth Barnhardt-Israel was able to be with them and pray with them during these last days of his life. Jon went home to be with the Lord shortly thereafter. Jon and his mother knew for certain, with total peace, he was stepping over into eternity from this life into the loving arms of his Savior, the Lord Jesus Christ, every bit whole.

Topic Discussion Question:

What is the biggest area of challenge for you that keeps you from being in peace and entering into rest?

Suggested Closing Prayer:

Lord God, we thank you that you are our shield from the storms of life. Heavenly Father, we thank you that after our flesh is destroyed we will see you, God, with our own eyes, and not another. How our heart yearns for you, Lord. Thank you, God, that we give every care to You, because You care for us. In Jesus' mighty name. Amen.

Additional Follow-Up Scriptures:

Job 19:26–27	And after my skin has been destroyed, yet in my flesh I will see God NIV
2 Corinthians 12:7–9	Three times I pleaded with the Lord to take it away from me. But he said to me, "My grace is sufficient for you, for my power is made perfect in weakness." NIV
Psalms 63:1	O God, you are my God, earnestly I seek you. NIV

Notes:

_____

_____

_____

Rev. Lillian Elizabeth Barnhardt-Israel

listen|imagine|view|experience

AUDIO BOOK DOWNLOAD INCLUDED WITH THIS BOOK!

In your hands you hold a complete digital entertainment package. In addition to the paper version, you receive a free download of the audio version of this book. Simply use the code listed below when visiting our website. Once downloaded to your computer, you can listen to the book through your computer's speakers, burn it to an audio CD or save the file to your portable music device (such as Apple's popular iPod) and listen on the go!

How to get your free audio book digital download:

1. Visit www.tatepublishing.com and click on the elLIVE logo on the home page.
2. Enter the following coupon code:
   3bbb-86da-ab3a-788f-268a-3a8a-8857-5c47
3. Download the audio book from your elLIVE digital locker and begin enjoying your new digital entertainment package today!